Isis M. Atallah

Neurofibromatosis type 1 tumourigenesis

Isis M. Atallah

Neurofibromatosis type 1 tumourigenesis

Identifying new genes involved in malignant transformation

Südwestdeutscher Verlag für Hochschulschriften

Impressum/Imprint (nur für Deutschland/only for Germany)
Bibliografische Information der Deutschen Nationalbibliothek: Die Deutsche Nationalbibliothek verzeichnet diese Publikation in der Deutschen Nationalbibliografie; detaillierte bibliografische Daten sind im Internet über http://dnb.d-nb.de abrufbar.
Alle in diesem Buch genannten Marken und Produktnamen unterliegen warenzeichen-, marken- oder patentrechtlichem Schutz bzw. sind Warenzeichen oder eingetragene Warenzeichen der jeweiligen Inhaber. Die Wiedergabe von Marken, Produktnamen, Gebrauchsnamen, Handelsnamen, Warenbezeichnungen u.s.w. in diesem Werk berechtigt auch ohne besondere Kennzeichnung nicht zu der Annahme, dass solche Namen im Sinne der Warenzeichen- und Markenschutzgesetzgebung als frei zu betrachten wären und daher von jedermann benutzt werden dürften.

Coverbild: www.ingimage.com

Verlag: Südwestdeutscher Verlag für Hochschulschriften GmbH & Co. KG
Heinrich-Böcking-Str. 6-8, 66121 Saarbrücken, Deutschland
Telefon +49 681 37 20 271-1, Telefax +49 681 37 20 271-0
Email: info@svh-verlag.de

Approved by: Berlin, Humboldt Universität, Diss., 2009

Herstellung in Deutschland (siehe letzte Seite)
ISBN: 978-3-8381-3447-5

Imprint (only for USA, GB)
Bibliographic information published by the Deutsche Nationalbibliothek: The Deutsche Nationalbibliothek lists this publication in the Deutsche Nationalbibliografie; detailed bibliographic data are available in the Internet at http://dnb.d-nb.de.
Any brand names and product names mentioned in this book are subject to trademark, brand or patent protection and are trademarks or registered trademarks of their respective holders. The use of brand names, product names, common names, trade names, product descriptions etc. even without a particular marking in this works is in no way to be construed to mean that such names may be regarded as unrestricted in respect of trademark and brand protection legislation and could thus be used by anyone.

Cover image: www.ingimage.com

Publisher: Südwestdeutscher Verlag für Hochschulschriften GmbH & Co. KG
Heinrich-Böcking-Str. 6-8, 66121 Saarbrücken, Germany
Phone +49 681 37 20 271-1, Fax +49 681 37 20 271-0
Email: info@svh-verlag.de

Printed in the U.S.A.
Printed in the U.K. by (see last page)
ISBN: 978-3-8381-3447-5

Copyright © 2012 by the author and Südwestdeutscher Verlag für Hochschulschriften GmbH & Co. KG and licensors
All rights reserved. Saarbrücken 2012

To my husband and my son,

To my mother, my father, my sister

To my family

To my friends

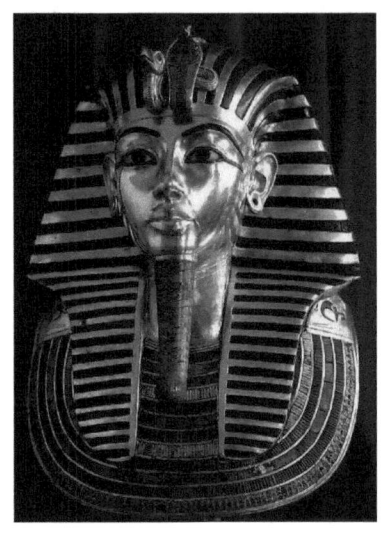

*It was an old tradition, passed on from Egypt into Greece,
that a God hostile to men's peace and quiet
was the inventor of the Sciences.*

J.J. Rousseau
Discourse on Arts and Sciences

Acknowledgements

I walked a long way before writing this thesis. During this walk I was not alone; I felt the support of several persons whom I would like to thank today for helping me to achieve a dream.

My love for research was a gift from my father. He fostered my interest for science, medicine and languages already in my childhood. I want to thank my mother because she gave me the strength and the support to achieve this doctoral thesis, and my sister for always being by my side. I want to thank all my family and friends: Jesús García, Amalia y Oliva Mantecón, Lucrecia Apolinario, Isabel Quirós, Javier Arnáiz and Víctor Román for their help and love.

I would like to express my eternal gratitude to Fernando de la Cruz and Javier León, my teachers and tutors of the Medical Faculty of the Cantabria University who, even though I was only 17 years old, believed in me and helped me to take my first steps in research. I also would like to thank Prof. Phillip Halban, Dolores de la Fuente and Peter Nürenberg, because they encouraged me to investigate and allowed me to accumulate all kind of experiences. Very special thanks go to the Asociación Cántabra para las Neurofibromatosis, especially to Ramón and Conchi for allowing me to participate with them in discovering neurofibromatoses. Furthermore, I am thankful to the Asociación Juvenil de Intercambios de Estudiantes and the COIE of the Cantabria University for their economic support.

I want to thank especially my supervisor Nikola Holtkamp for helpful discussions and help with manuscripts, but also for her patience, her availability and her friendship. I would like to express my eternal gratitude to Prof. von Deimling, whose vast knowledge, expertise, understanding, and patience considerably contributed to my graduate experience. Very special thanks go to Christian Hartmann for his computer assistance and his friendship. I want also to acknowledge David Reuß, Anastasia Afanassieva, Stefan Blumensath, and Jens Burucker for sharing their knowledge with me and Jana Mucha and Kathrein Stichling for their technical support. I want to thank Ingeborg Küchler who provided me with statistical advice and María Angeles Vega, Ingmar Rupp and Robert O'Dowd for helping me with translations.

To finish, this doctoral thesis would have not been possible without the financial support of the Berliner Krebsgesellschaft and I would like to express my eternal gratitude to this foundation, especially to Barbara Fey and Beate Eichenberg for their kindness.

Table of contents

ACKNOWLEDGEMENT 3
TABLE OF CONTENTS 5
LIST OF ABBREVIATIONS 9
LIST OF FIGURES 12
LIST OF TABLES 14
Abstract
    English 15
    German 17
    Spanish 19
    French 21

1   Introduction
    1.1 Neurofibromatosis type 1 23
        1.1.1 Epidemiology 23
        1.1.2 History 23
        1.1.3 NF1-diagnostic features 24
        1.1.4 NF classification 28
        1.1.5 NF1-associated tumours 30
            1.1.5.1. Neural crest tumours 30
            1.1.5.2 Non-neural crest malignancies 32
        1.1.6 Histopathology of NF1-associated peripheral nerve sheath tumours 33
        1.1.7 Genetics of NF1 34
        1.1.8 Neurofibromin 34
        1.1.9 Actual knowledge about NF1-associated tumourigenesis 36

2 Aims of the Project.. 39

3 Material and Methods

3.1 Material 40
3.1.1 Machines... 40
3.1.2 Chemical products 41
3.1.3 Antibodies... 44
3.1.4 Buffers and solutions 45
3.1.5 Fungible material 47

3.2 Methods 48
3.2.1 Tumour samples.. 48
3.2.2 Microarray hybridisation 50
3.2.3 Western blotting... 53
3.2.4 Immunohistochemistry 56
3.2.5 Immunofluorescence.. 57
3.2.6 Single-strand-conformational-polymorphism 58
3.2.7 DNA-sequencing 62

4 Results

4.1 Gene expression analysis: Microarray hybridisation............ 66
4.2 Verification on the protein level 69
4.2.1 MMP-13 expression.. 69
4.2.2 P53 expression 70
4.2.3 Syndecan 71
4.2.3.1. Syndecan-1 72
4.2.3.2 Syndecan-4 73

4.2.4 Platelet derived growth factor receptor alpha 76
4.2.5 Prion protein 76
4.2.6 Proteolipid protein 76
4.2.7 Matrilin-2 77
4.2.8 Apolipoprotein-D 78
4.3 MMP-13 and p53 80
4.3.1 Is MMP-13 expression induced by mutant p53? 80
4.3.2 Relevance of MMP-13 expression and *TP53* status in MPNST patients 83
    4.3.2.1 Clinical description of the MPNST patients 83
    4.3.2.2 Clinical relevance of MMP-13 expression and p53 status in MPNST patients 84

5   Discussion

5.1 Gene identification: Microarray hybridisation 87
5.2 Verification on the protein level 91
5.2.1 MMP-13 and p53 92
    5.2.1.1 MMP-13 92
    5.2.1.2 p53 93
    5.2.1.3 Is MMP-13 expression induced by mutant p53? 94
    5.2.1.4 Clinical relevance of MMP-13 expression and p53 sequence alterations in MPNST patients 96
5.2.2 Syndecan 98
    5.2.2.1 Syndecan-1 99
    5.2.2.2 Syndecan-4 100
5.2.4 Platelet derived growth factor receptor alpha 101
5.2.5 Prion protein 103
5.2.6 Proteolipid protein 104
5.2.7 Matrilin-2 105

   5.2.8 Apolipoprotein-D 106

6 Conclusions 108

7 Bibliography……………………………………………………..…...112

List of Abbreviations

A	Ampere
AA	Acrylamide
ApoD	Apolipoprotein D
APS	Amoniumpersulfate
bp	Basepair
BSA	Bovine serum albuminates
CHROM	Chromogen substrate
°C	Degree Celsius
ddH2O	Double distilled water
dH2O	Distilled water
dNF	Dermal neurofibroma
dNTP	Deoxynucleoside triphosphate
ECL™	Enzymatic chemioluminutesescence, Amersham Pharmacia Biotech (Freiburg)
EDTA	Ethylenediaminutesetetraacetic acid
EGFR	Epidermal growth factor receptor
EtBr	Ethidium bromide
g	Gram
h	Hour
HCl	Hydrochloric acid
H&E	Haematoxylin and Eosin
HEMA	Hematoxylin
HNO_3	Nitric acid
HP BK	Horse peroxidase blocking reagent

HPF	High power field
HRP	Horseradish Streptavidin Peroxidase
IHC	Immunohistochemistry
IF	Immunofluorescence
kDa	Kilodalton
kb	Kilobase
µl	Microliter (10^{-6}L)
mA	Milliampere (10^{-3}A)
mg	Milligram (10^{-3}g)
$MgCl_2$	Magnesium chloride
min	Minute
ml	Milliliter (10^{-3}L)
MMP-13	Matrix metalloproteinase 13
MPNST	Malignant peripheral nerve sheath tumour
mtr-2	Matrilin-2
NaCl	Sodium chloride
NF	Neurofibroma
NF1	Neurofibromatosis type 1
PBS	Phosphate buffered saline
PCR	Polymerase chain reaction
PDGFR-α	Platelet derived growth factor receptor alpha
PLP	Proteolipid protein
pNF	Plexiform neurofibroma
PNS	Peripheral nervous system
PrP	Prion protein
r.p.m.	rotations per minute
RT	Room temperature
sec	Second
SDS	Sodium dodecyl sulfate

List of Abbreviations

SSCP	Single-strand conformational polymorphism
SSH	Suppression subtractive hybridisation
Syn	Syndecan
TEMED	Tetramethylethylendiamin
TBE	Tris-borate-EDTA
TRIS	Tris-(hydroxymethyl)-aminomethane
T-TBS	Tween®-20 and tris buffered saline
UV	Ultraviolet
V	Volt
vNB	virtual Northern blot
W	Watt
WB	Western blot

List of Figures

Figure 1: Tilesius' drawings of "Wart man" 24
Figure 2: Clinical diagnostic features of a patient with Neurofibromatosis type 1 26
Figure 3: Neurofibromatosis type 1 radiographic features 27
Figure 4: Histopathological characteristics of NF1-associated tumours 33
Figure 5: Model of NF1-associated tumourigenesis 37
Figure 6: Schematic representation of the aims of the project 39
Figure 7: Schematic representation of the methods performed 48
Figure 8: Microarray assay 52
Figure 9: RNA quality verification 66
Figure 10: Heat map and histological features of the tumours 68
Figure 11: Western blot for MMP-13 69
Figure 12: MMP-13 immunofluorescence 70
Figure 13: Western blot for p53 70
Figure 14: p53 immunohistochemistry 71
Figure 15: Syndecan- 1 immunohistochemistry 72
Figure 16: Western blot for syndecan-4 73
Figure 17: Syndecan- 4 immunohistochemistry 74
Figure 18: Western blot for PDGFR-alpha 76
Figure 19: Western blot for prion protein 76
Figure 20: Western blot for proteolipid protein 77
Figure 21: Western blot for Matrilin-2 77
Figure 22: Western blot for Apolipoprotein D 78
Figure 22: *TP53* mutation analysis 81
Figure 24: Most common *TP53* mutation sites 82
Figure 25: Cumulative survival analysis for tumour location 83

Figure 26: Time until occurrence of metastasis in MPNST patient carrying the Pro^{72} allele.. 84

Figure 27: Role of Prion protein in apoptosis..104

Figure 28: Schematic representation of this doctoral thesis 110

Figure 29: New model of NF1-peripheral nerve tumourigenesis 111

List of Tables

Table 1: Diagnostic criteria for NF1 24
Table 2: Riccardi classification of typical and atypical neurofibromatoses 29
Table 3: Classification of segmental neurofibromatosis by Roth 29
Table 4: List of antibody dilutions for WB and IHC 44
Table 5: Definition of grading parameters for the FNCLCC system.................... 49
Table 6: Protocol to prepare a gel for Western Blot 54
Table 7: Acrylamide % and transfer duration depending on the protein size....... 55
Table 8: Template for protocol MSIP 57
Table 9: *TP53* primers and PCR conditions 60
Table 10: Silver staining protocol 62
Table 11: Results of syndecan-1 and syndecan-4 immunohistochemistry 75
Table 12: Western blot results 80
Table 13: *TP53* polymorphisms in MPNST patients 83
Table 14: Patient and tumour characteristics.. 86
Table 15: Genes identified to be differentially expressed in MPNST, pNFs and dNFs
.... 88
Table 16: *TP53* mutation analysis previously performed in MPNST.................. 95

Abstract

Neurofibromatosis type 1 (NF1) is one of the most frequent dominantly inherited diseases. The incidence is about 1:3,500 newborn. NF1 patients harbour an increased risk of developing benign nerve sheath tumours such as dermal neurofibromas (dNFs) and plexiform neurofibromas (pNFs) and a 10% lifetime risk of developing malignant peripheral nerve sheath tumours (MPNST). MPNST that usually arise from pre-existing pNFs are highly aggressive malignancies and have a dismal prognosis.

To identify genes involved in NF1-tumourigenesis we performed gene expression analysis applying cDNA array technology. 26 NF1-associated tumours and 2 MPNST cell cultures were examined. Using immunohistochemistry and/or Western blotting, 8 genes were evaluated on the protein level. Thus, *TP53* gene status was screened by single strand conformational polymorphism in 36 MPNST patients.

Expression of 57 genes differed significantly between dNFs, pNFs and MPNST. MMP-13, p53, Syn-1 and PDGFR-α were confirmed on the protein level to be overexpressed in MPNST while Syn-4, PrP and ApoD showed increased expression in neurofibromas. MMP-13 expression was significantly associated with p53 accumulation and with a higher risk of relapse in MPNST patients. *TP53* mutants were observed in 11% of MPNST patients. Polymorphism *TP53Pro^{72}* was associated with the development of metastases.

A panel of genes useful for subclassification of nerve sheath tumours was identified by expression analysis. NF1-associated and sporadic MPNST could not be distinguished by this approach. MMP-13, a matrix metalloproteinase involved in tumour invasion and dissemination, was reported to be stimulated by certain *TP53* mutants. The observation that most MMP-13 positive MPNST carried wild-type *TP53* suggests the existence of other regulation mechanisms. Nevertheless, MMP-13 expression might be considered a risk factor for relapse.

This doctoral thesis has identified several proteins likely to be involved in NF-1 tumourigenesis. The existence of medicines that inhibit MMP-13 and PDGFR-α expression might help to improve therapy for MPNST patients.

Zusammenfassung

Die Neurofibromatose Typ 1 (NF1) ist eine der häufigsten dominant vererbten Erkrankungen. Die Inzidenz liegt bei 1:3.500 Neugeborenen. Patienten mit NF1 haben ein erhöhtes Risiko gutartige Nervenscheidentumore wie dermale Neurofibrome (dNFs) und plexiforme Neurofibrome (pNFs) zu entwickeln und ein 10%iges Risiko im Laufe ihres Lebens an einem malignen peripheren Nervenscheidentumor (MPNST) zu erkranken. MPNST, die in der Regel aus pNFs hervorgehen, sind sehr aggressiv und haben eine schlechten Prognose.

Um Gene zu identifizieren, die eine Rolle bei der NF1-assoziierten Tumorgenese spielen, wurde eine Genexpressionsanalyse mittels cDNA-Array Technologie durchgeführt. 26 NF1-assoziierte Tumore und 2 MPNST Zelllinien wurden untersucht. 8 Gene wurden auf Proteinebene mittels Immunhistochemie und/ oder Western blot untersucht. Insgesamt wurden Tumore von 56 NF1 Patienten analysiert. Außerdem wurde das *TP53* Gen mittels single strand conformational polymorphism (SSCP) auf Mutationen untersucht.

Siebenundfünfzig Gene zeigten signifikante Expressionsunterschiede zwischen dNF, pNF und MPNST. Auf Proteinebene konnte eine stärkere Expression von MMP-13, p53, Syn-1 und PDGFR-α in MPNST nachgewiesen werden. Syn-4, PrP und ApoD zeigten erhöhte Expression in Neurofibromen. MMP-13 Expression korrelierte mit p53 Ablagerung und einem erhöhtem Rezidivrisiko. *TP53* Mutanten wurde nur in 11% der MPNST detektiert. Die p53Pro^{72} Variante zeigte eine Assoziation mit Metastasierung.

Die Studie identifizierte eine Serie von Genen, die bei der Subklassifizierung von Nervenscheidentumoren hilfreich sein können. NF1-assoziierte und sporadische MPNST konnten nicht differenziert werden. Frühere Studien zeigten, dass die Matrixmetalloproteinase MMP-13, welche eine Rolle bei Invasion und

Metastasierung spielt, durch p53 Mutanten stimuliert wird. Die Beobachtung, dass die Mehrheit der hier untersuchten MMP-13-positiven Tumore wildtyp *TP53* trugen, weißt auf andere Regulationsmechanismen. MMP-13 könnte sich allerdings als prognostischer Marker eignen.

Diese Doktorarbeit hat Proteine identifiziert, die mutmaßlich eine Rolle bei Entwicklung von Nervenscheidentumoren spielen. Bereits vorhandene Medikamente, die MMP-13 und PDGFR-α inhibieren, könnten zu verbesserter Behandlung von MPNST Patienten beitragen.

Resumen

La neurofibromatosis tipo 1 (NF1) es una de las enfermedades autosómicas dominantes más frecuentes. Su incidencia es de 1 por cada 3.500 nacimientos. Los pacientes con NF1 tienen un mayor riesgo de desarrollar tumores benignos de la vaina de los nervios periféricos tales como los neurofibromas cutáneos (dNFs) o plexiformes (pNFs) y un riesgo del 10% de desarrollar a lo largo de su vida un tumor maligno de la vaina de los nervios periféricos (MPNST). Los MPNST, suelen desarrollarse generalmente a partir de un pNF preexistente, son tumores muy agresivos y de muy mal pronóstico.

Para identificar los genes implicados en la formación de tumores associados a la NF1 realizamos un análisis de expresión de genes aplicando tecnología de cDNA microarrays. Se examinaron 26 tumores primarios associados a la NF1 así como 2 cultivos celulares de MPNST. Usando técnicas de inmuhistoquímica y/o Western blotting se examinó la expresión a nivel protéico de 8 genes. Se analizaron tumores de 56 pacientes. Además se escrutó el gen *TP53* en busca de mutaciones por polimorfismo conformacional de cadena simple.

Cincuenta y siete genes mostraron diferencias de expresión entre las 3 entidades tumorales dNFs, pNFs y MPNST. A nivel protéico, se confirmó la sobreexpresión de MMP-13, p53, Syn-1 y PDGFR-α en MPNST mientras que la expresión de Syn-4, PrP y ApoD estaba aumentada en neurofibromas. La expresión de MMP-13 se asocia de forma significativa a la acumulación de p53 y a un mayor riesgo de recidiva. Se encontraron mutaciones en *TP53* en 11% de los MPNST. El polimorfismo *TP53Pro^{72}* mostró estar asociado a enfermedad metastásica.

Este estudio ha identificado una serie de genes útiles en la subclasificación de los tumores la vaina de los nervios periféricos. No se encontraron diferencias entre los MPNST esporádicos y los asociados a la NF1. Estudios previos mostraron que MMP-

13, una metaloproteasa de la matriz involucrada en los procesos de invasión y metástasis, era estimulada por mutantes de *TP53*. La observación de que la mayoría de los tumores positivos para MMP-13 expresan la forma salvaje de *TP53* sugiere la presencia de otros mecanismos reguladores. Sin embargo, la expresión de MMP-13 puede considerarse como factor de riesgo de recidiva.

Esta tesis doctoral ha contribuído a la identificación de varias proteínas involucradas en la formación de los tumores asociados a la NF1. La existencia de medicamentos que inhiben la expresión de MMP-13 y PDGFR-α podrán mejorar el tratamiento actual de los pacientes con MPNST.

Resumé

La Neurofibromatose type 1 (NF1) est l'une des maladies autosomiques dominantes parmi les plus fréquentes. Son incidence affecte à 1 sur 3.500 nouveau-nés. Les patients avec la NF1 ont un risque accru de développer des tumeurs bénignes de la gaine des nerves périphériques comme les neurofibromes dermales (dNFs) et plexiformes (pNFs) et un risque de par vie de 10% de développer une tumeur maligne de la gaine des nerves périphériques (MPNST). Les MPNST, qui surviennent normalement à un pNF pré-existant, sont des tumeurs très agressives avec un pronostic très sombre.

Pour identifier les gènes impliqués dans la formation des tumeurs associées à la NF1 on a analysé l'expression des gènes en utilisant la technologie cDNA. 26 tumeurs associées à la NF1 et 2 cultures cellulaires de MPNST ont été examinées. En faisant usage des techniques d'immunohistochimie et/où Western blotting 8 gènes ont été examinés au niveau protéique. Les tumeurs de 56 patients ont été analysées. Aussi, on scruta le gène *TP53* à la recherche de mutation par polymorphisme de conformation des simples brins.

Les niveaux d'expressions de 57 gènes ont différé significativement entre les 3 entités tumorales: dNFs, pNFs et MPNST. Au niveau protéique, MMP-13, p53, Syn-1 et PDGFR-α ont été confirmé d'être surexprimés dans les MPNST, tandis que les expressions de Syn-4, PrP et ApoD étaient augmentés dans les neurofibromes. L'expression de MMP-13 dans les MPNST s'associa significativement avec l'accumulation de p53 et un risque plus élevé de rechute des MPNST. Une mutation de *TP53* a été détectée dans 11% des patients avec MPNST. Le polymorphisme de *TP53Pro*^{72} montra une association signifiante avec le développement de métastases.

Cette étude a identifié une série de gènes utiles pour la subclassification des tumeurs de la gaine des nerves périphériques. Aucune différence d'expression n'a été observée entre les MPNST sporadiques et les associées à la NF1. D'antérieures études montrèrent que MMP-13, une matrix métalloprotéase impliquée dans les procès d'invasion et de métastase, était stimulée par des mutants de *TP53*. L'observation que la majorité des tumeurs exprimant MMP-13 portaient la forme sauvage de p53, nous suggére la présence d'autres mécanismes de régulation. Cependant, MMP-13 peut être considéré comme un facteur de riske de rechute.

Cette thèse doctorale a contribué à l'identification de plusieurs protéines qui jouent probablement un rôle dans la formation des tumeurs associées à la NF1. De plus, l'existence de médicaments capables d'inhiber la surexpression de MMP-13 et PDGFR-α pourra améliorer la thérapie des patients avec MPNST.

1 Introduction

1.1 NEUROFIBROMATOSIS TYPE 1

Neurofibromatosis type 1 (NF1), also called von Recklinghausen's neurofibromatosis and peripheral neurofibromatosis, is a term applied to a dominant inherited neurocutaneous disease caused by an alteration of the *NF1* gene mapping to chromosome 17q11.2.

1.1.1 EPIDEMIOLOGY

NF1 is one of the most common autosomal dominant inherited disorders with an estimated birth incidence of 1:2,500[1] and a prevalence of 1:3,500 individuals[2]. Though NF1 has a penetrance of almost 100%, an extreme variability even within the members of the same family is possible.

1.1.2 HISTORY

The name von Recklinghausen's neurofibromatosis comes from a monograph published in 1882 by von Recklinghausen on the 25th anniversary of the foundation of the Berlin Pathologic Institute, established by his mentor and the father of pathology, Rudolf Virchow. However, the earliest portrayal of a man with NF1 was found in a 13th century Syrian illustration and was attributed to a scribe named Heinricus. In 1768 the British Physician M. Akenside described a man who had

> "a constant succession of wens that shot out in several places, on his head, trunk, arms and legs; which indisposition he inherited from his father."

Another report "Case history of extraordinary unsightly skin" was made by Tilesius in 1793 and included several drawings in colour of a "Wart man" with multiple fibrous tumours (Figure 1).

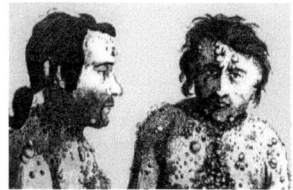

Figure 1: Tilesius' drawings of „Wart Man"

1.1.3 NF1-DIAGNOSTIC FEATURES

Diagnosis of NF1 is based on clinical criteria (Table 1) and is most commonly suggested by cutaneous features. The cardinal features of NF1 are café-au-lait macules, neurofibromas and Lisch nodules present in 95% of the patients. Café au lait macules (Figure 2; A) may be present at birth, but are not noticed in the first few months of life. There is no relationship between the number and localisation of café au lait spots and NF1 severity. Both axillary and inguinal freckling (Figure 2; A) develops in 70% of patients during the puberty and are highly specific for NF1. Lisch nodules (Figure 2; B) are multiple melanocytic

Table 1: Diagnostic criteria for NF1

The presence of two or more of the following signs identifies NF1 patients:
1. Six or more café au lait patches
- φ > 5mm in prepubertal
- φ > 15mm in postpubertal individuals
2. Two or more neurofibromas or one plexiform neurofibroma
3. Axillary or inguinal freckling
4. Two or more Lisch nodules
5. Optic nerve glioma
6. A distinctive osseous lesion with or without pseudoarthrosis:
- dysplasia of the sphenoid wing
- thinning of long bone cortex
7. A first-degree relative (parent, sibling or offspring) with NF1 according to the above criteria.

hamartomas of the iris (clumps of pigment cells). They usually appear in late childhood and do not impair vision. Their detection often confirms NF1 diagnosis in individuals having multiple café au lait spots. However, the clinical hallmark of the NF1 is the development of dermal neurofibromas (dNFs) and plexiform neurofibromas (pNFs). dNFs (Figure 2; B) most commonly appear in late childhood or adolescence as small spongy subcutaneous nodules. In contrast, pNFs usually are congenital and characterised by a large soft subcutaneous mass following the course of diffusely thickened peripheral nerves (Figure 2; D). pNFs may affect the skin and superficial muscle causing hypertrophy or deformation of the nearby tissue and diffuse hyperpigmentation of the overlying skin. They can transform into malignant peripheral nerve sheath tumours (MPNST).

Optic glioma and some osseous lesions are included as NF1 diagnostic criteria because their occurrence should suggest NF1. Optic gliomas are tumours made up of glial cells and may occur at any point of the optic nerve (Figure 3; C). Though optic gliomas are rarely malignant, they may cause painless proptosis, decreased visual acuity or neurological trouble. Bony abnormalities such as sharp scoliosis, dysplasia of a long bone (Figure 3; B) or the sphenoid wing may provide useful diagnostic clues. A very sharp focal deformity of the spine, due to vertebral dysplasia, is almost exclusive to NF1 (Figure 3; A).

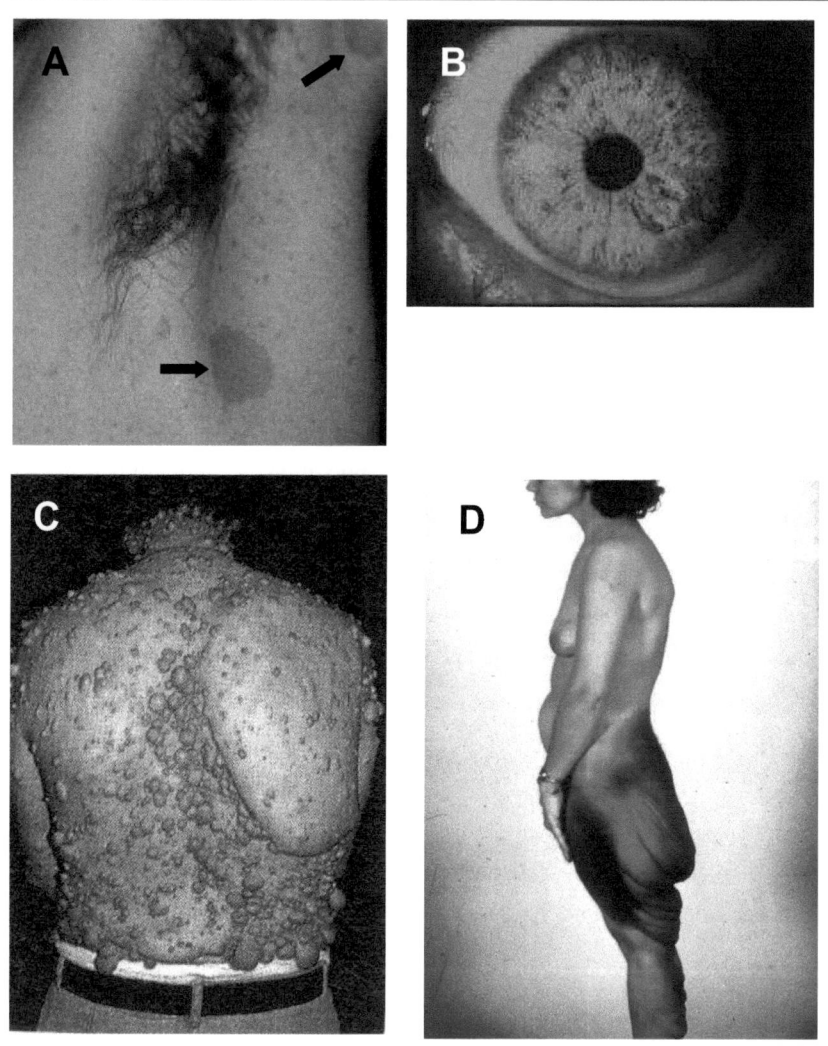

Figure 2: Clinical diagnostic features of a patient with neurofibromatosis type 1 A) Café au lait spots (arrow) and axillary freckling; B) Lisch nodules (hamartoma of the iris); C) Patient presenting several hundreds of nodular and polypoid dermal neurofibromas; D) Huge plexiform neurofibroma that infiltrates the lower back, buttock and proximal and distal lower extremities.

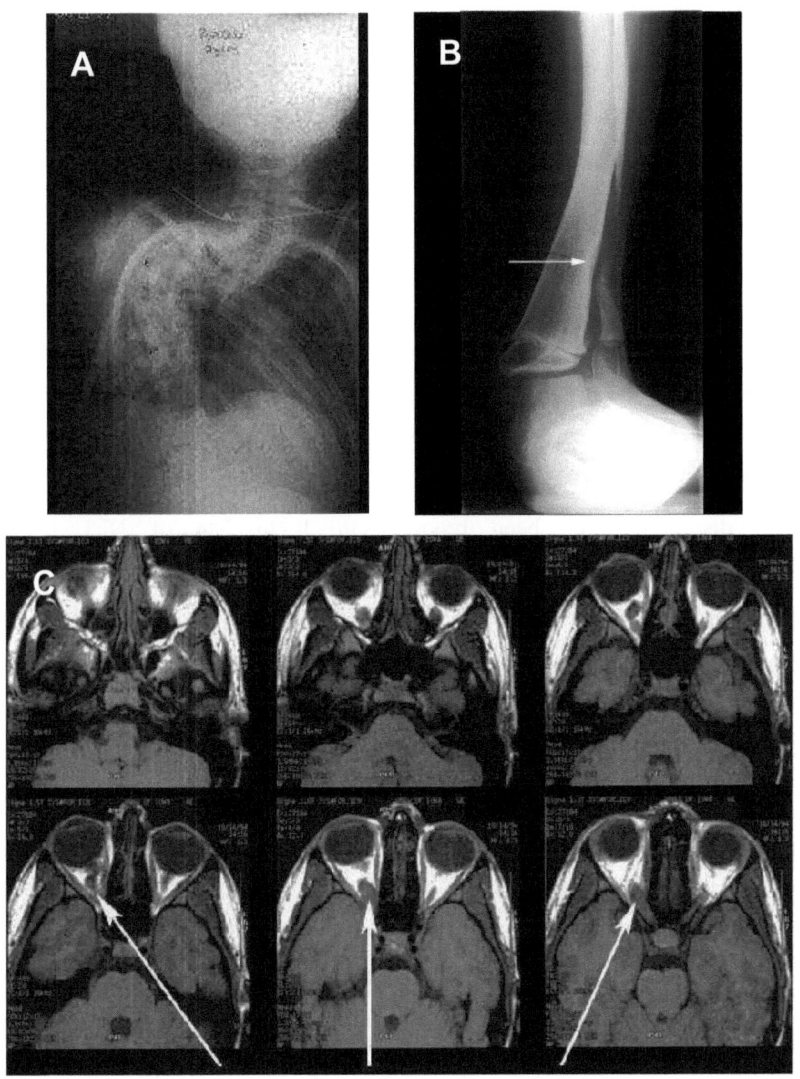

Figure 3: A) Radiograph of the cervical spine demonstrating a severe kyphotic deformity, characteristic of NF1. Posterior scalloping is present due to hypoplasia of the posterior elements. B) This radiograph shows an anterolateral bowing of the tibia and a lytic bone lesion with sclerotic margin (arrow); fibular pseudoarthrosis in a 10 year old male with NF1. C) T1-weighted RMI sagittal images demonstrate enlargement of the intraorbital and intracranial right optic nerve.

Other NF1 manifestations include abnormalities in the development of the central nervous system (CNS) such as megalencephaly or seizures. Evaluation of the brain is required to exclude a tumour as the cause of seizures. Hydrocephalus caused by aqueductal stenosis is one of the most frequent complications and produces symptoms related to abnormal intracranial pressure. Cognitive and learning disabilities have also been shown to be present in up to 80% of children with NF1 and have significant effects on their learning performance and everyday life[3]. The most common cognitive problems are with perception, attention, language and motor deficit.

Pulmonary manifestations such as interstitial fibrosis and bullae occur in 5 to 10% of NF1 patients. Interstitial fibrosis characteristically involves both lungs symmetrically with some basal predominance, whereas bullae usually are asymmetric and tend to develop in the upper lobes[4].

Endocrine disorders have been reported in 1 to 3% of NF1 patients. Pheochromocytoma is the most common disorder present in 1 to 6% of adults[5-7]. In contrast, central precocious puberty is seen in 2.5 to 6% [6, 8-10] of children, almost invariably caused by a tumour in the hypothalamus. Although short stature is observed in 13% of NF1 patients[10], growth hormone deficiency was found in only 2.5% of children with NF1[6].

1.1.4 NF CLASSIFICATION

Riccardi classified in 1982 the neurofibomatoses into eight different forms[11]. The most common type is the classic form (NF1). The NF2 describes bilateral acoustic neurinomas. Unusual combinations of features must be assigned to the remaining categories (Table 2). Type 5 corresponds to segmental NF and was defined by the presence of neurofibromas and/or café au lait spots with segmental distribution and without systemic involvement or family history. Segmental NF has an estimated frequency in the general population of 0.001[12]. The proposed mechanism is a mosaicism caused by a postzygotic somatic mutation affecting the NF1 gene in the primitive neural crest cells. The more premature the mutation arises in the developing embryo, the more generalised would be the phenotype.

Table 2: Riccardi classification of typical and atypical neurofibromatoses

Category	Description	Features
Type 1	Von Recklinghausen's disease	Multiple café au lait spots; Lisch nodules; neurofibromas
Type 2	Acoustic	Acoustic neurinoma (bilateral 90%)
Type 3	Mixed	Intermediate between the first two types
Type 4	Variant	Café-au-lait spots and neurofibromas; variable family history
Type 5	Segmental	Café-au-lait spots or neurofibromas in one unilateral segment
Type 6	Café-au-lait spots	Café-au-lait spots only
Type 7	Late onset	Onset of disease after age 30
Type 8	Not otherwise specified	Typical features of NF that do not fit into one of the above-mentioned categories

Because of the heterogeneity of NF, in 1987, Roth et al[13] proposed four different subgroups of the segmental type, according to unilateral or bilateral disposition, family history and systemic involvement (Table 3).

Table 3: Classification of segmental neurofibromatoses by Roth

Category	Description	Features
Type I	True segmental	Segmental café au lait spots and/or neurofibromas, no systemic involvement, non inherited
Type II	Localised with deep involvement	Segmental with deep systemic involvement, non inherited
Type III	Hereditary segmental	Segmental, no deep involvement, inherited
Type IV	Bilateral segmental	Bilateral segmental café au lait spots and/or neurofibromas, no deep involvement, non inherited

1.1.5 NF1-Associated Tumours

Predisposition to both benign and malignant tumour formation is one of the cardinal features of NF1.

1.1.5.1 Neural Crest Tumours

Neural crest tumours associated with NF1 occur in both central and peripheral nervous systems and together account for a substantial portion of the medical presentation of NF1.

Dermal neurofibromas

Dermal neurofibromas (dNFs) are benign tumours that arise in peripheral nerves at any site and appear in 95% of NF1 patients. Although dNFs are well defined and do not infiltrate surrounding tissues, they can grow to a nodular or polypoid mass of an enormous size. dNFs rarely impair nerve function but may cause problems due to their location. Their major impact is usually cosmetic and they can be removed surgically, although regrowth sometimes occurs. Growth of dNFs commonly occurs in association with puberty and pregnancy.

Plexiform neurofibromas

Plexiform neurofibromas (pNFs) are usually congenital but continue to grow later in life. They occur in about 30% of NF1 patients and infiltrate long portions of nerves and surrounded tissue resulting in widespread disfigurement and mechanical complications. pNFs are not malignant, however up to 30% transform to MPNST[14]. The signs of malignancy are rapid growth of a portion of the tumour or the occurrence of pain.

Malignant peripheral nerve sheath tumour

MPNST are highly aggressive sarcomas, they are difficult do detect and are associated with poor prognosis[15]; the 5-year survival rate is only 21%[16]. MPNST involve large and medium nerves most commonly in the buttock, thigh, brachial plexus and paraspinal regions. In addition, they infiltrate surrounding tissues, relapse commonly after surgery and may metastasise early to lung, liver, brain, soft tissue, bone, regional lymph nodes, skin and retroperitoneum. Extremely rare in general population (incidence of 0.001%), MPNST arise in 8-13% of patients with NF1[16]. They generally develop in the third decade of life (28-36 years) in NF1 patients and in the fourth decade (40-44 years) of life in non-NF1 patients and are slightly more frequent in females.

Tumours of the Central Nervous System (CNS)

Tumours of the CNS are common in NF1. Most of them are gliomas and have usually a benign course and histology. However, some of them can show signs of malignancy such as rapid growth or invasion. Symptoms depend on their location and size and they can cause impaired vision, dysarthria, dysphagia, ataxia, megalencephaly and hydrocephalus.

Optic gliomas, generally pilocystic astrocitoma, account for 1/3 of the CNS tumours and occur in 14-15% of NF1 patients[17]. They are usually associated with ipsilateral exophthalmos and might produce strabismus and loss of vision which is sometimes difficult to detect in small children. Tumour progression in the first years of life can be followed by a spontaneous regression of the tumour as has been assessed by MRI[18].

Other NF1-associated brain tumours include astrocytomas of other cranial nerves(2%)[19] and more rarely intracerebral schwannoma[20], ganglioglioma[21], meningiomas[22] and medulloblastomas[23, 24]. Another CNS manifestation of NF1 is the so-called "unidentified bright object" or UBO, which is a lesion with increased signal on a T2 weighted sequence of an MRI examination of the brain. These UBOs are typically found in the cerebellar peduncles, pons, midbrain, globus pallidus, thalamus, and optic radiations. Their exact identity remains a mystery since they disappear over time (usually, by the age of 16). They might represent a focally degenerative piece of myelin.

Spinal tumours are considered one of the most usual complications of NF1. They are usually benign but they may compress not only the nerve roots but even the spinal cord itself. They can be detected by MRI in 36-38% of NF1 patients[25, 26]. However, only 5-7% of patients will present symptoms such as pain, weakness, muscular atrophy and hyperreflexia.

Other neural crest tumours

Neuroblastoma, a pediatric tumour of immature nerve cells, is rarely observed in NF1 patients. Pheochromocytoma, on the other hand is strongly associated with NF1. Although extremely rare in the normal population, 1 to 6% of the NF1 patients develop pheochromocytomas[5-7]. This tumour arises from chromaffin cells of the adrenal medulla and can produce significant hypertension, perspiration, headache, unexplained anxiety and flushing[7]. Other tumours derived from neural crest cells associated with NF1 are the malignant cutaneous or uveal melanoma[27-30] and the medullary carcinoma of the thyroid[7].

1.1.5.2 Non- Neural Crest Malignancies

Children with NF1 are predisposed to develop leukaemia. Although leukaemia is the most common malignancy in childhood, the distribution of leukaemia subtypes differs between NF1 children and the normal population[31, 32]. Chronic and acute myeloid leukaemias as well as myelomonocytic leukaemia or myeloproliferative disease were found to be associated with NF1[33]. Furthermore, rhabdomyosarcoma has been reported to occur in 1% of NF1 patients[34], especially in the first years of life. Wilms tumour has also been linked to NF1, though the association is very weak.

Less than 1% of NF1 patients will develop a Wilms tumour[35] which normally appears in the first months of life or in adolescence.

1.1.6 HISTOPATHOLOGY OF NF1-ASSOCIATED PERIPHERAL NERVE SHEATH TUMOURS

dNFs are either nodular or polypoid. They consist of a mixture of cell types, including Schwann cells, perineural-like cells and fibroblasts embedded in a matrix of collagen fibers and mucosubstances. On hematoxylin and eosin stained sections they appear as well-circumscribed but non-encapsulated spindle cell tumours submerged in a large amount of extracellular material. The nuclei of the spindle cells are characteristically curve- or S-shaped and the faintly eosinophilic wavy fibers seen within the tumour are reticulin positive. They are mostly in the dermis but may extend into the subcutaneous fat.

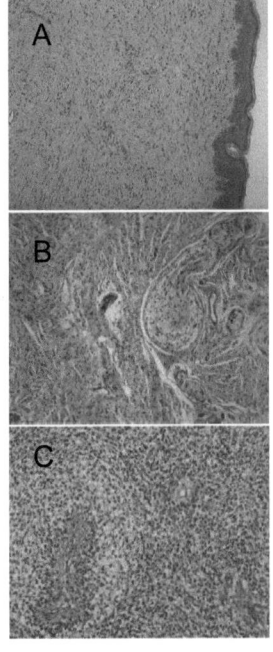

pNFs are neurofibromas of large nerve fibers. Their diffuse and soft nature is often compared to 'a bag of worms'. Histologically they appear as globules of neural tissue. The globules represent enlarged, tortuous plexi of Schwann cells and axons embedded in a mucinous stroma within a thickened perineurium. They usually show interlaced bundles of elongated cells with wavy nuclei without atypism associated with wire-like strands of collagen.

Figure 4: Histopathological characteristics of NF1-associated tumours: A) dNF; B) pNF; C) MPNST

MPNST typically show a fasciculated growth of tightly packed cells with abundant faintly eosinophilic cytoplasm and elongated nuclei. Positive immunostaining for p53 and for Ki-67/MIB-1 (proliferation marker) is present in the majority of tumours[36]. Furthermore, 50-70% MPNST express S100 (marker for neuroectodermal cells). However, S100 expression, a calcium binding protein, is not specific for MPNST. Antibody to S100 stains also ependymomas, astrogliomas, Langerhans cells and almost all benign and malignant melanomas and their metastases.

Although NFs and MPNST normally show drastic differences in histopathological features, sometimes it may be difficult to distinguish between borderline tumours. This may pose not only diagnostic but also therapeutic challenges.

1.1.7 GENETICS OF NF1

NF1 is a monogenic disorder caused by the inactivation of the *NF1* gene in one allele. Approximately 50% of NF1 patients carry a "de novo" mutation in the *NF1* gene. It is noteworthy that the *NF1* is among the human genes with the highest mutation rate, $1\text{-}2 \times 10^4$ gametes per generation, 10 times more than the average[37]. Interestingly, 80% of the "de novo" mutations are due to the inactivation of the paternal allele[38, 39]. However, no association was observed between the paternal age and the mutation incidence[40]. On the other hand, *NF1* total or partial deletions occur in 5-10% of cases and are usually observed in the maternal chromosome[41-43]. NF1 is also a pleiotropic disease, because a single gene mutation has several different consequences in different tissues of the organism.

1.1.8 NEUROFIBROMIN

The *NF1* gene was identified in 1990 and mapped on chromosome 17q11.2. It is one of the largest human genes, composed of 60 exons spanning over 350 kb of genomic DNA. It encodes a large cytoplasmic protein named neurofibromin (2818 amino acids) which has a role in tumour suppression[14]. One of the functions of neurofibromin is to reduce cell proliferation by accelerating the inactivation of Ras, which plays a pivotal role in mitogenic intracellular signalling pathways[44]. Neurofibromin has a GAP-related domain that interacts with Ras and mediates hydrolysis of GTP- (active) to GDP- (inactive) Ras. The domain responsible for GAP (GTPase activating protein) activity spans only 10% of neurofibromin and little is known about the additional functions of its other domains. However, the important role of this highly conserved protein (60% amino acid homology between drosophila and human neurofibromin) is underlined by the observation that $NF1^{-/-}$ mice are not viable[45].

Studies in Drosophila have suggested that neurofibromin also has non-Ras-GAP functions that involve regulation of intracellular cAMP[46]. *NF1* mutant flies are smaller in body size and this phenotype can be rescued by overexpression of protein kinase A but not by manipulating Ras signalling[47]. These results suggest that some of the NF1 clinical abnormalities, such as short stature, may result from other, yet unknown functions in specific cell types.

An association of neurofibromin and microtubules has been demonstrated by double labelling immunofluorescence and confocal microscopy[48]. The region of neurofibromin involved in this interaction was shown to reside within the NF1-GAP related domain[49]. Previous experiments have demonstrated that monomeric tubulin can impair the ability of neurofibromin to interact with Ras[49]. The functional significance of the association of neurofibromin and microtubules is still unknown; however, it may place neurofibromin in a readily accessible subcellular compartment where it can be efficiently recruited to regulate Ras. Interestingly, neurofibromin is in stable association with kinesin-1[50], a protein involved in the transport of protein complexes, organelles and mRNA to specific destinations in an ATP- and microtubules-dependent manner[51, 52]. Therefore, the association of NF1 and kinesin-1 suggests a new function for neurofibromin in the transport of vesicular cargoes within the cells. Thus aberrant transport of neurotransmitter could affect the development of the cerebral cortex and might explain the learning disabilities and cognitive problems related to patients with NF1 mutations[53-55]. Additionally, neurofibromin was observed to bind all 4 members of the mammalian syndecans. Neurofibromin forms a complex with Syndecan and CASK, which have overlapping subcellular distributions[56] and might be important for the subcellular localisation of neurofibromin and Ras inactivation.

1.1.9 ACTUAL KNOWLEDGE ABOUT NF1-ASSOCIATED TUMOURIGENESIS

It is now accepted that tumour formation is the result of multiple sequential mutations in key genes. A germinal inactivation of one *NF1* allele (generally, a point mutation) leads to NF1[14]. Following Knudson's model[57], a somatic second hit inactivation of the other allele leads to loss of functional neurofibromin and subsequent development of many types of tumours.

dNFs are the most common tumour type in NF1. Several studies over the past few years have demonstrated at the DNA, RNA and protein level that the neoplastic cell origin in NFs is the Schwann cell[58, 59]. Furthermore, recent studies suggest that $NF1^{+/-}$ cells contribute to neurofibroma formation, and that factors produced by $NF1^{+/-}$ cells might be important for facilitating or accelerating tumour development[60]. EGFR expression in transgenic mouse Schwann cells elicited features of NFs such as Schwann cell hyperplasia, excess collagen, mast cell accumulation and progressive dissociation of non-myelin forming Schwann cell axons[61]. Therefore, EGFR overexpression is thought to be an early event in NF1-tumourigenesis and malignant progression might require additional genetic lesions.

The difference in the mechanism of tumourigenesis between dNFs and pNFs is unclear. The amount of NF1 mRNA processing might play a role in determining which tumour develops, as dNFs have the lowest amount of mRNA editing, pNFs an intermediate amount and MPNST the highest quantity of NF1 gene editing[62].

As pNFs are normally congenital tumours, loss of functional neurofibromin is thought to occur in a Schwann cell precursor population. Furthermore, pNFs can undergo malignant transformation and form MPNST. Recently, *NF1* mutation spectrum analysis demonstrated that NF1 patients with large *NF1* deletions carried a higher lifetime risk of developing MPNST[63]. Recently, Levy et al identified 5 genes that might predict malignant progression of pNFs (MMP9, VEGFR3, TRAILR2, SHH and GLI1).

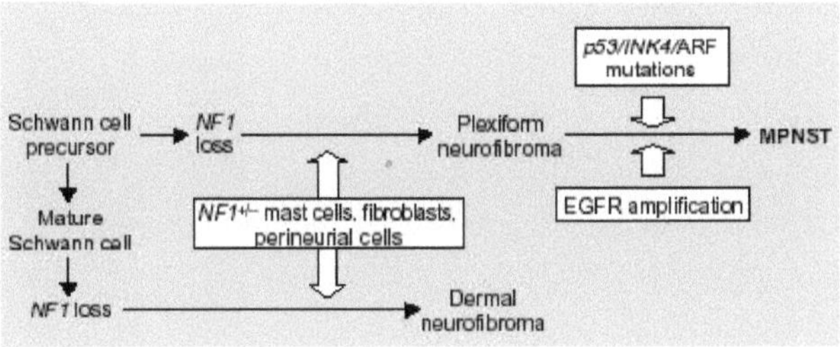

Figure 5: Model of NF1-associated tumourigenesis according to Dasgupta and Gutmann: *NF1* loss in Schwann cell precursors during development in cooperation with NF1$^{+/-}$ fibroblasts, perineural cells and mast cells results in pNF formation. The accumulation of other genetic changes promotes progression to MPNST. *NF1* loss in mature Schwann cells in cooperation with NF1$^{+/-}$ cells possibly results in dNF formation.

Several alterations in important mitogenic and cell-cycle regulatory pathways were found to synergise with *NF1* loss to undergo malignant transformation. Mutations in tumour suppressor genes such as *TP53*[65, 66], or at the *CDKN2A* locus affecting both $p16^{INKa}$ and $p14^{ARF}$[67] have been identified in MPNST. Similarly, a loss of expression of another cell-cycle growth regulator, $p27^{Kip1}$, has also been reported[68]. EGFR was found to be overexpressed in primary MPNST, MPNST cell lines and some S100+ Schwann cells in primary NFs[69]. Furthermore, EGFR-amplification was observed in 26% of human MPNST[69, 70]. It is noteworthy that brain lipid protein was observed to be expressed by a subpopulation of EGFR-positive NF1$^{-/-}$ mutant Schwann cells suggesting that it regulates Schwann cell-axon interaction[71]. Moreover, elevated

CD44 expression in MPNST cells was shown to be at least partially dependent on EGFR overexpression and to contribute to a more invasive behaviour[72].

2 Aims of the Project

Until now, only a few genetic alterations have been identified to be involved in tumour formation of NF1-associated peripheral nerve sheath tumours. Molecular mechanisms involved in tumourigenesis are still largely unknown. In order to bring more light into the process of malignant transformation of nerve sheath tumours, the Institute of Neuropathology performed Suppression Subtractive Hybridisation (SSH) with a pNF and an MPNST and identified, prior to my arrival, 133 genes with differential expression. To gain further insight into the molecular pathogenesis involved in tumour formation or progression of nerve sheath tumours, it was planned to:

1. Identify genes differentially expressed in dNFs, pNFs and MPNST applying the cDNA microarray technology and validate previous results in a larger panel of tumours.
2. Verify on the protein level the expression of some gene candidates selected based on functional criteria such as a relation to malignancy or clinical relevance by immunohistochemistry and/or Western blotting.
3. Assess the clinical and functional relevance of the differential expression by review of the literature and statistical analysis when possible.

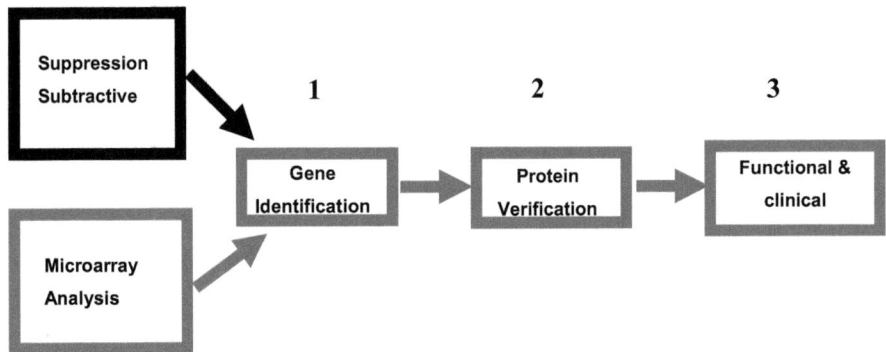

Figure 6: Schematic representation of the aims of the project. Framed in blue are the phases of the project in which I was involved.

3 Material and Methods

3.1 MATERIAL

3.1.1 MACHINES

Agitator	SM-30, Edmund Bühler (Hechingen)
Cassettes Radiographic	Cronex® DuPont (Wilmington)
Casting stand	Mini-PROTEAN®II Bio-Rad (Munich)
Centrifuge	Biofuge fresco Heraeus Kendro (Hanau)
	Macrofuge 1.OR Heraeus Kendro (Hanau)
Computer	Satellite 1110-Z20, TOSCHIBA (Neuss)
Cryo-microtome	HM 560 MICROM (Walldorf)
Digital-camera	C-5050 Zoom, Olympus (Hamburg)
Electrophoresis Power Supply	EPS 3501x2 Amerscham Pharmacia Biotech (Freiburg)
Electrophoresis chamber SSCP	Blue Sequ. Serva (Heidelberg)
Electrophoresis chamber agarose	E-92, Biometra (Göttingen)
Gel dryer	Serva (Heidelberg)
Heating block	SHT 100D, Bibby Stuart Scientific (Stone, Great Britain)
Homogenizer	Ultra-turrax® 125 basic, IKA®-Werke, (St Augustin)
Magnet agitator	L32, LABINCO (Merseburg)
Mixer	REAX Top, Heidolph (Kelheim)
Paraffin-microtome	HM 335E, Microm (Walldorf)

Microwave	Bosch (Stuttgart)
pH-meter	HI 9321, Hanna Innit (Kehl)
Pipetboy	Accu-jet®, BRAND (Wertheim)
Pipets	P10, P20, P100, P200, P1000 Gilson (Bad Camberg)
Power Supply	Power all 5000V, Serva (Heidelberg)
Protean II	xi | XL Vertical Electrophoresis Cells, Bio-Rad (Munich)
Sequence Editor	Version1.3, Applied Biosystems (Weiterstadt)
Sequencer	377, Applied Byosystems (Weiterstadt)
Stereo microscope	Leica/leitz DMRB (Bensheim) BX 50F with photo applicator, Olympus (Hamburg)
Thermocycler	Unoblock, Biometra (Göttingen)
Thermomixer	L32 Labinco (Merseburg)
Robot Immunostaining	Techmate™ 500/1000, DAKO (Hamburg)
Ultrasound waterbath	SONOREX RK31, Bandelin (Berlin)
UV Spectrophotometer	Ultrospec 2000, Pharmacia Biotech (Freiburg)
Vacuum	Greifenberg Antriebstechnik GmbH, (Markredwitz)
Waterbath	ETS-D4, IKA®-labor technique (St Augustin)
Weighing machines	SBC 51 and 33, SCALTEC (Heiligenstadt)
X-ray film processor	45 Compact PROTEC (Großgeschwenda)

3.1.2 CHEMICAL PRODUCTS

Acetone	Merck (Darmstadt)
Acetic Acid	Merck (Darmstadt)
Agarose	Sigma (Deisenhofen)

Antioxidant	Invitrogen (Leek, Netherlands)
Alconox®	J.T. Baker (Deventer, Netherlands)
Big Dye	PRISM® DyeDeoxy Terminator Cycle Kit, Applied Biosystems (Weiterstadt)
Bromphenolblue	Sigma (Deisenhofen)
BSA	Sigma (Deisenhofen)
ChemMate™ System Kit	Peroxidase/DAB, DAKO (Hamburg)
Chloroform	J.T. Baker (Deventer, Netherlands)
Deoxycholat	U.S.B. (Bad Homburg)
DNA extraction Mini Kit	QIAamp. Qiagen (Hilden)
DNA marker	PUC19 DNA /Msp 1 (Hpa II) Marker 23, Fermentas (St. Leon-Rot)
ECL™	Amersham Pharmacia Biotech (Freiburg)
EDTA	Sigma (Deisenhofen)
Eosin	Chroma (Münster)
Ethanol	Merck (Darmstadt)
Ethidium bromide	Serva (Heidelberg)
Extravidin®	Sigma (Deisenhofen)
Formamid	Fluka (Deisenhofen)
Ficoll-400	Sigma (Deisenhofen)
Gel Extraction Kit	QIAquick. Qiagen (Hilden).
Glycerol	Sigma (Deisenhofen)
Glycin	Merck (Darmstadt)
HCl	Merck (Darmstadt)
Hematoxylin	Merck (Darmstadt)
Isopropyl alcohol	Merck (Darmstadt)
Iso-pentan	Sigma-Alldrich (Seelze)
Liquid nitrogen	Leine & Linde (Berlin)

LDS Sample Buffer (4x)	NUPAGE Invitrogen (Leek, Netherlands)
Milk powder	Roth (Karlsruhe)
Methanol	Sigma (Deisenhofen)
Milk powder	Roth (Karlsruhe)
Nitrocellulose membrane	Trans-Blot® Bio-Rad (Munich)
Nonidet P-40	Boeringer (Mannheim)
Oligonucleotides	TP53 primers exon 1 to11 MWG Biotech (Ebersberg)
Protease inhibitor cocktail	Roche (Mannheim)
PCR Master Mix	Promega (Mannheim)
PCR Buffer	Promega (Mannheim)
PCR $MgCl_2$	Promega (Mannheim)
PCR dNTP	Promega (Mannheim)
PCR Taq polymerase	Promega (Mannheim)
Ponceau Rot	Merck (Darmstadt)
Protein marker	MagicMark™ Western Standard. Invitrogen (Leek, Netherlands)
Protein marker	Biotynilated SDS molecular weight standard mixtures. Sigma (Deisenhofen)
RNA Marker Template Mix	0.1-1Kb Novagen (Darmstadt)
Sample Reducing Agent (10x)	NUPAGE, Invitrogen (Leek, Netherlands)
SDS	Sigma (Deisenhofen)
Sodium citrate	Merck (Darmstadt)
Temed	Sigma (Deisenhofen)
TRIS	Trizma®Base, Sigma (Deisenhofen)
Trizol® Reagent	Total RNA Isolation Reagent, Gibco BRL (Heidelberg)
Tween®-20	Bio-Rad (Munich)
Urea	Sigma (Deisenhofen)

Water RNAse free	Aqua ad injectabilia, Braun (Melsungen)
Xylencyanol	Sigma (Deisenhofen)
Xylene	Sigma (Deisenhofen)
Xylol	J.T. Baker (Diventa, Netherlands)

3.1.3 ANTIBODIES

Table 4: List of antibody dilutions for WB and IHC.

1st Antibody	Dilutions WB	Size kDa	2nd Antibody	Dilutions IHC / IF	Pretreatment
Anti-ApoD	1:400	29	Mouse		
Anti-β-Actin	1:5,000	42	Mouse	1:1,000	without
Anti-Matrilin 2	1:100	125	Rabbit		
Anti-MMP-13	1:250	48, 54	Mouse	1:50	Microwave
Anti-p53	1:300	53	Mouse	1:100	Microwave
Anti-PDGFR-α	1:200	185	Rabbit	1:100	Microwave
Anti-PLP	1:500	26	Mouse		
Anti-prion serum Rabbit	1:300	25 unglyc.	Rabbit	1:100	Microwave
Anti-prion 3F4	1:3,000	25 unglyc.	Goat		
Anti-syndecan 1	1: 200	200, core 70	Maus	1:200	Microwave
Anti-syndecan 4	1: 100	220, core 35	Goat	1:100	without
2nd Antibody					
Anti-Goat-Biotin	1:3,000	-	-	1:1,000	-
Anti-Mouse-Biotin	1:1,000	-	-	1:300	-
Anti-Mouse IgG-peroxidase	1:2,000	-	-	-	-
Anti-Rabbit-Biotin	1:100	-	-	1:100	-
Anti-Rabbit IgG-peroxidase	1:10,000	-	-	-	-

First antibodies

Anti-apolipoprotein D	36C6, Novo Castra (Newcastle U.K.)
Anti-β-Actin	Sigma (Deisenhofen)
Anti-matrilin 2 serum	kindly provided by Dr. Raimund Wagener (Köln)
Anti-MMP-13	AB-4, Oncogene (Bad Soden)
Anti- proteolipid prot.	plpc1, Serotec (Düsseldorf)
Anti-p53	DO-7, DAKO (Hamburg)
Anti-PDGFR-α	C-20, Santa Cruz Biotechnologie (Heidelberg).
Anti-prion 3F4	kindly provided by Michael Baier, Robert-Koch Institute (Berlin)
Anti-prion serum rabbit	kindly provided by Michael Baier, Robert-Koch Institute (Berlin)
Anti-syndecan 1	CD138, BD Biosciences PharMingen (Heidelberg)
Anti-syndecan 4	N-19, Santa Cruz Biotechnologie (Heidelberg)

Second antibodies

Anti-Goat-Biotin	Chemicon AP106B (Hofheim)
Anti-Mouse-Biotin	Dako E0354, DAKO (Hamburg)
Anti-Mouse IgG-perox.	Amersham Biosciences NA931 (Freiburg)
Anti-Rabbit-Biotin	Dako E0353, DAKO (Hamburg)
Anti-Rabbit IgG-perox.	Amersham Biosciences NA934 (Freiburg)

3.1.4 BUFFERS AND SOLUTIONS

30% Acrylamide/bis	(37, 5:1) 29.2 g acrylamide + 0.8 g N,N'-bis-methylene-acrylamide + dd$H_2$0 to 100ml
Acetic acid SSCP	10 % acetic acid in ddH_2O
Blocking Buffer WB	5 g dry milk to T-TBS 0.5%

Developer SSCP	3 % Na_2CO_3 + 2.5 ml formaldehyde in 5,000 ml ddH_2O
Diffusion buffer	0,5 M amoniumacetate + 10 mM magnesiumacetate + 1mM EDTA + 0.1% SDS
Ethanol X%	X ml C_2H_5OH in 100 ml ddH_2O
Loading Buffer DNA	0.25% bromphenolblue + 0.25% xylencyanol + 15% ficoll-400 in ddH_2O; diluted 2:5 before use
Loading Buffer SSCP	45 ml formamide 90% + 5 ml 10x TBE + 100 µl EDTA 1mM + 0.005 g SDS 0.01% + 0.25 g bromophenolblue 0.25% + 0.125 g xylencyanol 0.25%
Loading Buffer sequencing	Formamide 90% / 50 mM EDTA-solution (5:1) (pH 8.0)
Lysis buffer	0.350 g NaCl + 0.4 g nonidet P40 + deoxycholate 0.2 g + ddH_2O to 40 ml + protease inhibitor cocktail
Nitric acid SSCP	1% HNO_3 in ddH_2O
PBS	20 g NaCl + 0.5 g KCl + 3.5 g $Na-H_2PO_4xH_2O$ + 0.5 g NaOH + ddH_2O to 2.500ml, pH=6.7
Protease inhibitor cocktail	1 tablet protease inhibitor cocktail in 2 ml ddH_2O
Running buffer WB	3.02 g Tris-Base + 14.2 g glycine + 0.1% SDS + ddH_2O to 1,000 ml, pH 8.3
Running buffer FA	20 ml 37% formaldehyde + 100 ml 10x FA gel buffer + 880 ml RNase free water
SDS 0.1%	1 g SDS in ddH_2O to 100 ml
Sephadex column	55 g sephadex in 750 µl ddH_2O pro column
Silver nitrate SSCP	2 g $AgNO_3$ in 2.000 ml ddH_2O
Transfer Buffer WB	3.0 g Tris-base + 14.4 glycin + 0.1% SDS + 200 ml methanol + ddH_2O to 1.000 ml, pH 8.3
TBS	8 g NaCl + 1.21 g Tris + ddH_2O to 1.000ml, pH 7.3

TBE	10.8 g Tris + 5.5 g boric Acid + 40 ml EDTA 0.5 M + ddH$_2$O to 1.000 ml
Tris-HCL 1.5 M, pH 8.8	18.15 g Tris base + ddH$_2$O to 100ml. Adjust pH with HCl
Tris-HCL 0.5 M, pH 6.8	6 g Tris Base + ddH$_2$O to 100ml. Adjust the pH with HCl
T-TBS 0.5%	500 µl Tween®-20 in 1.000 ml TBS

3.1.5 FUNGIBLE MATERIAL

Combs	Bio-Rad (Munich)
Cuvette-photometer	Sarstedt (Nümbrecht)
Cryo-tubes	Cryovial 4 ml, Roth (Karlsruhe)
Filter paper	Schleicher and Schuell (Dassel)
Glass plates WB	Outer 3/1mm & Short 5, Mini PROTEAN 3, Bio-Rad (Munich)
Glass-cover	Menzel (Braunschweig)
Latex gloves	Kimberly-Clark (U.S.A.)
Lumi-Film	Chemoluminescent detection film. Roche (Manheim)
Pasteur-pipette	One use, Sarstedt (Nümbrecht)
Pipet tips	Gilson (Bad Camberg)
Save-lock tubes	0.5 ml, 1.5 ml, 2 ml, Eppendorf (Hamburg)
Slides	Capillary gap microscope slides ChemMate™, DAKO (Hamburg)
	SuperFrost® Plus, Langenbrinck (Emmerdingen)

3.2 METHODS

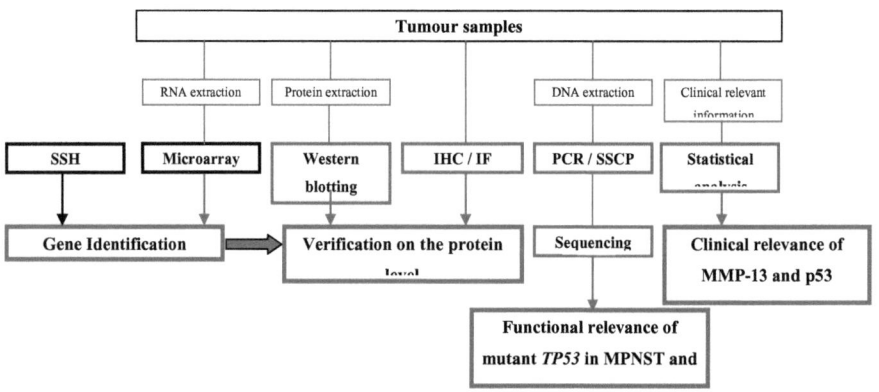

Figure 7: Schematic representation of the methods employed. Boxes framed in blue indicate steps that I have personally performed. SSH: Suppression subtractive hybridisation; IHC: immunohistochemistry; IF: immunofluorescence; PCR: Polymerase chain reaction; SSCP: Single strand conformational polymorphism.

3.2.1 TUMOUR SAMPLES

We collected 69 primary tumours: 46 MPNST, 9 pNFs and 14 dNFs from 56 patients at:

- University Eppendorf Hospital (Hamburg, Germany): 24 MPNST, 3 pNFs, 9 dNFs
- Robert-Rössle Hospital, Berlin (Germany): 11 MPNST
- Otto-von-Guericke University (Magdeburg, Germany): 5 MPNST
- Charité-Virchow Hospital, (Berlin, Germany): 6 MPNST, 6 pNFs and 5 dNFs

49 tumours were embedded in paraffin and 20 were frozen material (conserved at -80°C). Extracted DNA from 5 sporadic MPNST was provided by the Otto-von-Guericke-University. MPNST cell lines S462 and ST88-14 (kindly provided by Dr. Andreas Kurtz, Robert-Koch-Institute) were also analysed. Cell line S462 was

established from MPNST 24472. Clinical information was available for 36 MPNST patients. 22 MPNST originated from patients diagnosed with NF1 according to the NIH diagnostic criteria[73]. Second surgery after clinical progression was defined as recurrence. The investigations were carried out with informed consent. Following initial diagnosis in local neuropathologies, all tumour samples were reviewed by the same pathologist. Tumour histology was graded according to the Fédération Nationale de Centres de Lutte contre le Cancer (FNCLCC) system. Defining parameters are given in Table 5.

Table 5: Definition of grading parameters for the FNCLCC system

Parameter	Criteria
Tumour differentiation	
Score 1	Sarcomas closely resembling normal adult mesenchymal tissue
Score 2	Sarcoma for which the histologic typing is certain
Score 3	Embryonal and undifferentiated sarcomas; sarcoma of uncertain type
Mitosis count	
Score 1	0-9/10 HPF
Score 2	10-19/10 HPF
Score 3	≥20/10 HPF
Tumour necrosis	
Score 0	No necrosis
Score 1	≤50% Tumour necrosis
Score 2	<50% Tumour necrosis
Histologic grade	
Grade 1	Total score 2, 3
Grade 2	Total score 4, 5
Grade 3	Total score 6, 7, 8

HPF: high-power field

Further clinical information of MPNST patients is available in Table 14. Before DNA and RNA extraction and preparation of lysates each piece of tumour was stained with haematoxylin and eosin and examined histologically.

3.2.2 MICROARRAY HYBRIDISATION

Microarray hybridisation is a screening method for detection of differentially expressed genes. We performed cDNA microarray analysis to screen for differences in gene expression among MPNST, pNFs and dNFs and to verify in a larger panel of tumours the 539 genes that were identified in previous projects by SSH[74].

This technique was performed through the collaboration of several colleagues of the Institute of Neuropathology, including myself, Scienion and the Institute of Biochemistry, Charité University Hospital. Although I described briefly the full process, my personal role was limited to carrying out the RNA-DNA extraction of the tumour samples as well as the RNA quality verification by agarose gel.

RNA-DNA extraction by Trizol®

The tumour tissues were weighed and pulverised using a mortar and pestle. The tissue powder was further treated with a homogenizer. The samples were homogenised in 1 ml Trizol per each 100 g tissue and incubated 5 min at RT. 0.2 ml chloroform was added per ml Trizol reagent. The tubes were closed, shaken vigorously for 15 sec and incubated 3 min at RT. Afterwards, the samples were centrifuged at 3,000 rpm (Megafuge 1.OR Heraeus) for 10 min. Following the centrifugation, the mixture separated into a lower red, organic phase, an interphase, and a colourless upper aqueous phase. RNA remains in the aqueous phase, while the DNA remains in both organic and interphase.

RNA extraction: the aqueous phase was transferred to a new tube and mixed with 0.5 ml isopropyl alcohol per ml Trizol reagent. The samples were incubated 10 min at RT and centrifuged at 3.000 rpm for 10 min. The supernatant was removed. The RNA pellet was washed in 1 ml 75% ethanol per ml Trizol reagent. The samples were then vortexed and centrifuged 5 min at 2,000 rpm. The supernatant was removed once more and the RNA pellet was allowed to air-dry briefly before being resuspended in RNAse free water.

DNA extraction: the DNA was precipitated by adding and mixing 0.3 ml of 100% ethanol per 1 ml Trizol reagent to the supernatant. The samples were incubated 3 min at RT and centrifuged 5 min at 3,000 rpm. The supernatant was carefully removed and the DNA was washed twice in a solution containing 0.1 M sodium citrate and 10% ethanol. At each wash, the DNA pellet was stored in the washing solution for 30 min at RT. Following these 2 washes, the DNA pellet was resuspended in 1.5 ml 75% ethanol per ml Trizol reagent, stored for 3 min at RT and centrifuged at 2,000 rpm for 5 min at 4°C. The supernatant was then removed and the pellet was allowed to air-dry before being resuspended in ddH$_2$O. All steps of centrifugation were carried out at 4°C with the Megafuge 1.OR Heraeus Kendro Centrifuge.

DNA and RNA quality was checked in a 2% and 1.2% agarose gel, respectively, and adjusted to a volume of 6 µl with ddH$_2$O. 1 µg RNA was mixed with 2 µl RNA loading buffer. DNA PCR products were mixed 1:2 with DNA loading buffer.

Microarray construction and hybridisation

cDNA labelling and microarray hybridisation were performed at Scienion AG (Berlin). RNA quality was checked with a 2100 Bioanlyser by assessing the 28S/18S rRNA ratio at Scienion. 26 tumours (10 MPNST, 7pNF and 9 dNFs) from 24 patients fulfilled the quality criteria of intact RNA, which is essential for valid results. cDNAs were obtained from the RNAs by performing RT-PCR with oligo(dT)12-18 and aminoallyl modified dUTPs. Tumour cDNAs were then purified and coupled with Cy3 monoreactive NHS-ester (green). A reference cDNA was coupled with Cy5 monoreactive NHS-ester (red).

Arrays carrying 539 cDNAs fragments previously identified by SSH, 17 NF1-relevant genes (*TGFB1, MET, TP53, CDKN2A, CDKN2D, MKI67, HRAS, KRAS2, SDC4, CDKN1B, SAC, NF1, NF2, GAP43, CDH13* and *EGFR*) and 2 housekeeping genes (*GAPD* and *ACTB*) were constructed. Finally, the 558 resulting cDNAs were spotted in duplicates on coated slides and hybridised with the 26 tumour cDNAs and the reference cDNA at 42°C for 16h.

Microarrays were scanned with two wavelengths for Cy3 (570nm) and Cy5 (660nm) using a laser fluorescent scanner (GenePix 4000B scanner; Axon instruments, Union city, CA). The fluorescence intensity of each spot was quantified and fluorescence levels of the local background were subtracted.

Evaluation of Array Data

Evaluation of Array Data was performed at the Biochemistry Institute of the Humboldt University using the GeneSpring software package (Silicon Genetics, Redwood City, USA). Genes whose signals were too low were excluded. The 106 genes that produced proper signals were clustered hierarchically using an algorithm developed by Eisen (M. Eisen, http://rana.lbl.gov./EisenSoftware.htm). After elimination of doublets and candidates whose standard deviation was too high, 57 genes with significantly differential expression remained.

Figure 8: Microarray hybridisation: A) Microarray assay scheme; B) Scanned microarray after hybridisation

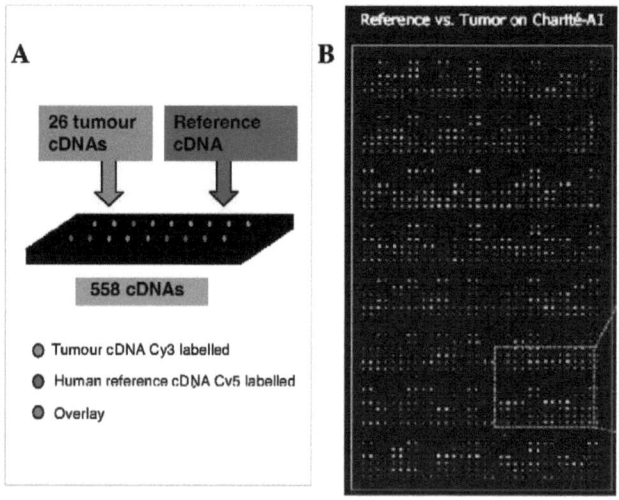

3.2.3. WESTERN BLOTTING

In order to verify the differential gene expression on the protein level, Western blotting (WB) was performed. By WB, proteins are size-fractionated in a polyacrylamide gel prior to being transferred to a nitrocellulose membrane for probing with an antibody. This technique allows detection of the expression patterns, quantity and size of the proteins.

Lysate preparation

Lysate preparation was performed with frozen material from 6 MPNST, 2 MPNST cell cultures, 6 pNFs and 4 dNFs. In order to prepare lysates from frozen tissue under optimal conditions it was necessary to work with equipment cooled with liquid nitrogen. Tumour samples were first pulverised using mortar and pestle. The tissue powder was then transferred to a 2 ml cup. Two ml lysis buffer was then added and vortexed. The samples were homogenised for 2 min by bath sonification and vortexed again prior to being spun (4°C, 10 min, 3.000 rpm; Megafuge 1.0R Heraeus). The supernatant was transferred to a 15 ml tube. The pellet was resuspended in 1 ml lysis buffer, homogenised by bath sonification, vortexed and centrifuged. The supernatant was added to the 15 ml tube. Lysates from cortex, placenta and gliomas were also prepared and used as controls for Western blotting. The protein concentration was determined by mixing 20 µl of the lysate in 1.5 ml 4:1 ddH2O-Bio-Rad protein assay reagent, vortexing and waiting 15 min. 1 ml from the solution was introduced into the spectrophotometer (Absorption 595 nm) to obtain the optic density of the solution and calculate the protein concentration using a reference curve.

The reference curve was obtained by performing a series of 10 different dilutions of BSA in dH$_2$0 (0.1µg/µl to 1µg/µl) and mixing in a tube 100 µl of each dilution with 2.5 ml dH$_2$0-Protein Biorad assay mixture (4:1) previously filtered. The tubes were vortexed and incubated for 15 min at RT. Afterwards 1 ml of each solution was introduced into the spectrophotometer (Absorption 595 nm) and optic densities were measured. The optic densities values obtained for each dilution were used to draw a curve that served as a reference to calculate the protein concentration of a tumour lysate from the optic density value.

Gel Casting

Cassettes were constructed by joining the outer and shorter glasses (previously washed with soap, and cleaned with ethanol 70%) and held by the Mini-PROTEAN®II casting stand. Resolving gel was prepared (Table 6), poured into a gel cassette to the top of the label tape and immediately overlaid with dH_2O. Incubation for 45 min allowed polymerization. The dH_2O was removed. Stacking gel was then prepared (Table 6) and poured into the gel cassette. A gel comb (with 10 teeth) was placed and after 30-45 min the gel was ready to be used.

Table 6: Protocol to prepare a gel for Western blot

	Stacking Gel 4%	RESOLVING GEL		
		7.5%	12%	X%
30% Acrylamide	1.32 ml	2.5 ml	4.0 ml	0.33x Xml
0.5 M Tris-HCl, pH 6,8	2.52 ml	-	-	-
1.5 M Tris-HCl, pH 8,8	-	2.5 ml	2.5 ml	2.5 ml
10% SDS	100 µl	100µl	100µl	100µl
ddH2O	6 ml	4.85 ml	3.35 ml	7.35-(0.33x X) ml
TEMED	10 µl	5 µl	5 µl	5 µl
10% APS	50 µl	50 µl	50 µl	50 µl
Total Volume	10 ml	10 ml	10 ml	10 ml

Western blotting

Tumour protein concentration was first adjusted to β-actin levels. Homogenates (protein + 5 µl Sample Buffer (4x) + 2 µl reducing agent (10x) + dH2O up to 20 µl) were denatured for 10 min at 70°C and loaded in the gel pockets. Reducing agent was added to reduce disulfide bonds and to generate monomers. The internal and external chambers were filled with running buffer. Additionally, 500 ml antioxidant was added to the internal chamber. Gel electrophoresis was performed under the following conditions: 100-115 mA per gel, 200 V and 100 W for 50 min.

Table 7: Percentage of acrylamide and transfer duration depending on the protein size

Protein <60 kDa	12% acrylamide gel	60 min transfer
Protein 60-140 kDa	10% acrylamide gel	75 min transfer
Protein >140 kDa	7.5% acrylamide gel	90 min transfer

After electrophoresis, proteins were blotted to a nitrocellulose membrane at 170 mA, 35 V and 100 W. The internal chamber was filled with transfer buffer and the external chamber with ddH$_2$0. The duration of the transfer depended on the protein size and the acrylamide gel concentration (Table 7). Afterwards, the transfer efficiency was examined by visualization of fractioned proteins with Ponceau red. Nitrocellulose membranes were incubated in Ponceau red for a few sec and transferred proteins became visible. The membranes were then washed in dH$_2$0 and T-TBS 0.5% and blocked for 60 min in blocking buffer. Membranes were then incubated overnight at 4°C with the first antibody and washed the next morning in T-TBS. All washing steps were performed in T-TBS 0.5% (3 times briefly, twice for 10 min). Incubation with the second antibody was performed for 60 min. If non-peroxidase-labelled second antibodies were used, an extra- incubation step with extravidin-peroxidase for 60 min was carried out. Visualization was performed with enhanced chemiluminescence (ECL). The membranes were incubated 1 min with ECL and placed into a cassette. The following steps were performed in a dark room. A lumi-film was laid over the membrane. The exposure time depended on the antibody used and varied from a few sec to 60 min. The film was developed using the x-ray film processor 45 Compact from PROTEC (Großgeschwenda).

3.2.4 IMMUNOHISTOCHEMISTRY

Immunohistochemistry (IHC) allows the study of the expression pattern and localisation of a protein within the histological context of a tissue (e.g. expression in tumour cells, nuclear or cytoplasmatic staining). Frozen tissues and paraffin-embedded materials can be used for IHC.

Tumour slide preparation

Paraffin-embedded tumours were cut into slices of 2-3 µm and frozen samples into 4-6 µm slices. DAKO ChemMate™ Capillary Gap Microscope Slides were used for the DAKO TechMate™ 500 /1,000. Slides from frozen tumours were fixed with cold acetone for 10 min before undergoing additional steps.

Immunohistochemistry with DAKO automatic machine TechMate™ 500

IHC with DAKO TechMate™ 500 was performed for p53 (54 tumours), Syn-1 and Syn-4 (29 tumours). Paraffin sections were first incubated in an oven at 60°C for 60 min to fix the tissues to the slides. Slides were then deparaffinised by incubation in xylol for 15 min and in a row of basins with different ethanol concentrations (2x 100%, 96%, 80%, 70% and ddH2O). Afterwards, slides were incubated twice for 5 min in sodium citrate (pH= 6) in a microwave oven at 800 W. The exposure to heat and to a sodium citrate solution is designed to break protein cross-links and unmask the antigens and epitopes, thus enhancing the binding capacity of the antibodies. However, antibody retrieval must be established for each antibody and may differ.

Dako ChemMate™ Products:
- BUF1: Buffer 1.20ml
- BUF2: Buffer 2.20ml
- BUF3: Buffer 3.20 ml
- dH2O: "Water wash", 20 ml
- AB1: 1st Antibody, 350 µl
- AB2: 2nd Antibody, 350 µl
- HP BK: Peroxidase blocking reagent, 750 µl
- HSP: Streptavidin peroxidase, 350 µl
- CHROM: Chromogen substrate, 750 µl
- HEMA: Hematoxylin, 350 µl

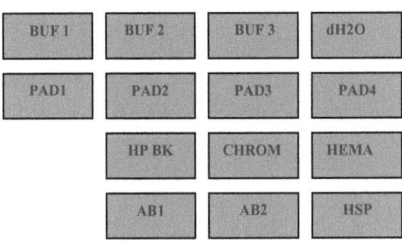

Table 8: Template for protocol MSIP

After cooling the sections for 20 min, the slides were arranged in pairs, face to face in an upright position in dH2O and placed in a DAKO ChemMate™ Holder for DAKO TechMate™ 500. The appropriate protocol was then run. The DAKO ChemMate™ System Kit Peroxidase/DAB and the template for protocol MSIP were used (Table 8). Slides were then dehydrated in graded alcohol and xylene prior to being coverslipped.

3.2.5 IMMUNOFLUORESCENCE

For immunofluorescence (IF) antibodies or antigens were labelled with fluorescent dyes. IF enabled us to visualize the subcellular distribution of a protein by fluorescence microscopy.

IF was performed for MMP-13 on 54 primary tumours: 36 MPNST and 9 pNFs and 9 dNFs.

Paraffin sections were deparaffinised by incubating the slides in an oven at 60°C for 15 min and dipping the slides twice in xylol for 10 min, alcohol 2x 100%, 96%, 80%, 70% and dH2O. The slides were then incubated in sodium citrate buffer (pH= 6; 3 times for 5 min at 600 W), cooled down and washed twice in PBS for 10 min. Afterwards, slides were blocked with a goat, rabbit or mouse normal serum mixture (dilution 1:10 in 3% BSA PBS) (same species as second antibody) for 30 min at RT and briefly washed. All washing steps were performed in PBS. Slides were then incubated with the first antibody (1:20-1:40) for 3-4 h in 200 µl PBS at RT, washed 3 times for 5 min and incubated with a Cy3-conjugated second antibody (dilution 1:100) for 1h at RT. Tumour slides were then washed and covered with glycerine. Slides were stored in darkness at 4°C until microscopic analysis.

3.2.6 SINGLE-STRAND CONFORMATIONAL POLYMORPHISM ANALYSIS (SSCP)

SSCP allows the identification of differences in nucleic acid sequences and is commonly used as a screening method for detecting mutations. It is based on the property of single-stranded DNA to fold up and form complex structures stabilised by weak intramolecular bonds. The electrophoretic mobility of nucleic acids in non-denaturating gels depends not only on their chain lengths but also on their conformation, which are dictated by the DNA sequence. Control samples must be run on the same gel so that differences from the wild-type pattern can be detected. SSCP is simple and sensitive but does not reveal the nature or position of the sequence alteration detected.

DNA extraction from paraffin slides and frozen slides
The QIAamp DNA Mini Kit was used for DNA isolation. For DNA extraction we used 10 slices (2-3 µm) from paraffin-embedded material and 30 thick slices (10µm) from frozen material. The tumour portion of the slides was grated and collected in a 1.5 ml cup. 180 µl buffer ATL and 40 µl proteinase K were added. The samples were then vortexed and incubated 1-3 h at 56°C and 750 rpm in a thermoblock (L32 Labinco). Afterwards, samples were briefly spun. Centrifugation steps were always 1 min at 13.000 rpm (Biofuge Fresco Heraeus Kendro Centrifuge). After adding 200 µl buffer AL, samples were vortexed, incubated at 70°C for 10 min and centrifuged

briefly. 200 μl ethanol was added. Samples were briefly vortexed and centrifuged. The supernatant was pipetted into a QIAamp Spin column placed in a clean 2 ml collection tube which has a filter membrane. 500 μl AW1 buffer was added. Samples were centrifuged and filtrates were discarded. 500 μl AW2 buffer was added to the QIAamp Spin column which was placed into a new tube. Samples were centrifuged once more and the flow-through was removed. To elute the DNA 50 μl buffer AE was poured onto a column which was placed into a new cup. DNA was eluted by centrifugation. This last step was performed twice.

DNA amplification: polymerase chain reaction (PCR)

PCR is a rapid and versatile in vitro method for amplifying defined target DNA sequences present within a source of DNA (for example genomic DNA). To permit such selective amplification, some prior DNA sequence information from the target sequence is required, enabling the construction of two oligonucleotide primer sequences (often 15-30 nucleotides long). These amplimers can initiate, in the presence of suitable heat-stable DNA polymerase and DNA precursors (dNTP), the synthesis of new DNA strands which are complementary to the individual DNA strands of the target DNA segment. Newly synthetised DNA strands then act as a template for further synthesis in subsequent cycles. DNA amplification is necessary to generate enough material for subsequent analysis.

Extracted tumour DNAs were diluted 1:20 in ddH$_2$O. The following reagents were used for PCR:

DNA	2 μl
MgCl$_2$ 25 mM	0.8μl (1mM); 1μl (1.25mM); 1.2 μl (1.5mM)
dNTP 40 mM	2 μl
PCR buffer	2 μl
Primer forwards (10 μM)	1 μl
Primer reverse (10 μM)	1 μl
Taq polymerase 100 units	0.4 μl (5 U/5 μl)
ddH2O	adjust to a final volume of 20 μl

Material and Methods

The Promega Master Mix containing polymerase, dNTP and $MgCl_2$ was used to amplify exon 3:

DNA	2 µl
Primer forwards (10µM)	1 µl
Primer reverse (10µM)	1 µl
Promega Master Mix	10 µl
ddH2O	6 µl

PCRs with *TP53* primers exon 1 to 11 (Table 9) were performed using the following conditions:

Table 9: *TP53* primers and PCR conditions

Exon	Primer sequence	Length	Temp.	$MgCl_2$
1 forward	5'-AAGTCTAGAGCCACCGTCCA-3'	234bp	53°C	1.5 mM
1 reverse	5'-ACCCCCAAACTCGCTAAGTC-3'	234bp	53°C	1.5 mM
2 forward	5'-ATCCCCACTTTTCCTCTTGC-3'	198bp	58°C	1.25 mM
2 reverse	5'-TCCCACAGGTCTCTGCTAGG-3'	198bp	58°C	1.25 mM
3 forward	5'-CATGGGACTGACTTTCTGC-3'	169bp	56°C	1.5 mM
3 reverse	5'-GGGACTGTAGATGGGTGAA-3'	169bp	56°C	1.5 mM
4_1 forward	5'-TGACTGCTCTTTTCACCCATC-3'	215bp	59°C	1.25 mM
4_1 reverse	5'-AGATGACAGGGGCCAGGAG-3'	215bp	59°C	1.25 mM
4_2 forward	5'-CTCCTGGCCCCTGTCATCT-3'	127bp	59°C	1.5 mM
4_2 reverse	5'-CCCCTCAGGGCAACTGAC-3'	127bp	59°C	1.5 mM
5_1 forward	5'-TTTGCCAACTGGCCAAGACC-3'	230bp	56.2°C	1 mM
5_1 reverse	5'-TCAGTGAGGAATCAGAGGCC-3'	230bp	56.2°C	1 mM
5_2 forward	5'-GTACTCCCCTGCCCTCAACAA-3'	301bp	60.9°C	1.25 mM
5_2 reverse	5'-TTCCACTCGGATAAGATGCTG-3'	302bp	60.9°C	1.25 mM
6 forward	5'-AGGCCTCTGATTCCTCACTGA-3'	199bp	55°C	1.25 mM
6 reverse	5'-AGAGACCCCAGTTGCAAACCC-3'	199bp	55°C	1.25 mM
7 forward	5'-GGCCTCATCTTGGGCCTGTG-3'	107bp	63°C	1.5 mM
7 reverse	5'-GTGTGCAGGGTGGCAAGTGG -3'	107bp	63°C	1.5 mM
8 forward	5'-AATGGGACAGGTAGGACCTG-3'	256bp	58.6°C	1.25 mM
8 reverse	5'-ACCGCTTCTTGTCCTGCTTG-3'	256bp	58.6°C	1.25 mM
9 forward	5'-CCTTTCCTTGCCTCTTTCCT-3'	173bp	59.4°C	1 mM
9 reverse	5'-CCACTTGATAAGAGGTCCCAAG-3'	173bp	59.4°C	1 mM
10 forward	5'-CTCCCCCTCCTCTGTTGCT-3'	149bp	58.2°C	1.25 mM
10 reverse	5'-AGGGGCTGAGGTCACTCAC-3'	149bp	58.2°C	1.25 mM
11 forward	5'-TGTCATCTCTCCTCCCTGCT-3'	142bp	60.9°C	1.25 mM
11 reverse	5'-CAGTGGGGAACAAGAAGTGG-3'	142bp	60.9°C	1.25 mM

The PCR-program used was:

94°C;	3 min	Initial denaturation
94°C;	40 sec	Denaturation
Primer Temp.;	30 sec	Annealing — 37 cycles
72°C;	40 sec	Extension
72°C;	10 min	Final extension

Agarose gel electrophoresis

A 2% agarose gel was prepared by mixing 2 g agarose with 0.6 x TBE to a final volume of 100 ml. The solution was then boiled in a microwave oven and cooled down shortly before adding 2 µl of ethidium bromide 100%. PCR products were mixed with loading buffer (1:1) and loaded to the solidified agarose gel. The DNA marker (Puc19) was used to determine the proper size of PCR products. Gels were run 15 min at 160 V and documented under UV light.

Single-Strand conformational polymorphism gel casting

SSCP glass plates were washed with soap, cleaned with ethanol 70% and impregnated with xylene prior to assembly. All *TP53* exons were analysed in a 14% AA 1:50 gel (24.01 ml acrylamide 40%, 9.8 ml bisacrylamide 2%, 7 ml 10x TBE, 3.5 ml glycerine and 13.77 ml ddH2O). The gel solution was mixed and poured between the 2 glass plates. A 40-tooth comb was then placed and the gel was allowed to polymerize for 90 min with a wet tissue over the comb to prevent drying out. After polymerization, gel plates were assembled on the SSCP-electrophoresis chamber. 1x TBE was used as SSCP running buffer.

Single-strand conformational polymorphism electrophoresis

PCR products were mixed with SSCP loading buffer (4:1), denatured for 10 min at 95°C and immediately cooled on ice. 4.5 µl of each sample was then loaded to a SSCP gel. SSCP electrophoresis was performed under the following conditions: 500 V and 6 mA for 18 h.

Silver staining

Gels were fixed in a frame prior to staining. The staining steps are listed in Table 10.

Table 10: Silver staining protocol

Solutions	Incubation times
10% Ethanol	10 min
1% Nitric acid	30 seconds
ddH$_2$O	1x wash
Silver nitrate	Minimum 20 min
ddH$_2$O	3x washed
Developer	Until bands are visible
10% Acetic acid	2 min
ddH$_2$O	1x wash

After staining, gels were laid on filter paper and dried in a gel-dryer at 80°C for 90 min.

3.2.7 DNA SEQUENCING

This method allows us to determine the exact nucleic acid sequence of a DNA region previously amplified.

DNA extraction from polyacrylamide gels

DNA bands showing a mobility shift were excised with a clean and sharp scalpel from the polyacrylamide gel and collected in 1.5 ml cups. 100 µl of diffusion buffer was added and the cup was incubated at 50°C for 30 min. After 1 minute of centrifugation (13,000 rpm, Biofuge fresco Heraeus Kendro centrifuge), the supernatant was carefully removed and passed to a new cup. 300 µl buffer QG was added and mixed. To bind the DNA, the sample was applied to a QIAquick column and centrifuged for 60 sec. The flow-through was discarded and 0.75 ml buffer PE was added to the column. The samples were centrifuged twice and the flow-through was rejected. The QIAquick column was then placed in a new cup. 50 µl buffer EB was added and the tubes were centrifuged to elute the DNA. To elute residual DNA, 30 µl additional buffer EB was added and the tubes were centrifuged again.

DNA reamplification: polymerase chain reaction

To reamplify DNAs extracted from SSCP gels, a PCR with the Promega master mix was used:

DNA	10 µl
Primer forward (10µM)	2.5 µl
Primer reverse (10µM)	2.5 µl
Promega Master Mix	25 µl
ddH2O	10 µl

The PCR-program explained in section 3.2.6 was carried out. PCRs quality and quantity were checked on a 2% agarose gel.

DNA purification

To purify DNA the Multiscreen®PCR Millipore plate was used. DNAs were poured in a 96-well plate and washed twice with 60 µl ddH$_2$O under vacuum conditions. DNAs were then resuspended in 30 µl ddH$_2$O and resolved for 10 min at 37°C. The quantity and quality of the purified DNA was checked on a 2% agarose gel.

Cycle sequencing

Cycle sequencing amplified one DNA strand by using fluorescent dNTPs (adenosine: green; thymidine: red; cytosine: blue and guanosine: black) allowing them to be detected by the semiautomated sequencer (model 373A; Applied Biosystems, Foster City, CA). The PRISM® DyeDeoxy Terminator Cycle Kit (Big Dye) was used to label the DNA:

DNA	5 µl to 7.5 µl depending on the DNA concentration
Big Dye	2 µl
Forward or reverse primer	0.5 µl

The PCR program used for amplification was:

95°C; 5 min	Initial denaturation	
95°C; 15 sec	Denaturation	
Primer temp.; 15 sec	Annealing	} 25 cycles
60°C; 4 min	Final extension	

Afterwards, the samples obtained from cycle sequencing were passed through a sephadex column in order to remove the excess fluorescent dNTPs. Sephadex columns were prepared mixing 55 mg sephadex G50 in 750 µl ddH$_2$O per column and centrifuged twice for 2 min at 3,000 rpm (Biofuge fresco Heraeus Kendro centrifuge) to remove the excess water. The samples were applied to the center of the sephadex column and centrifuged. The resulting flow-through was collected and evaporated at 70°C until all the liquid was gone.

Sequencing gel casting

Glass plates were thoroughly washed with Alconox®, rinsed with ddH$_2$O and dried carefully with colourless tissues. Glass plates were then assembled and clamped. Gel solution was poured between the plates, avoiding bubble formation, and a 36-tooth comb was placed on top. After polymerization (90 min) the gel was inserted into the sequencer. Protocol of the sequencing gel:

Acrylamid Bis 29:1	7.5 ml
Urea	18 g
1x TBE	6 ml
ddH$_2$O	23 ml
APS 10%	350 µl
TEMED	20 µl

Gel loading and electrophoresis

6 µl of DNA samples were mixed with 4 loading buffer, denaturised for 2 min at 95°C and immediately placed on ice. 1 µl per sample was loaded on a sequencing gel

and run at 2,500 V and 30 W. 1x TBE was used as running buffer. Resulting data were analysed by using the Sequence Editor Program, Version 1.3, and the Data Analysis Program, Version 1.2 from Applied Biosystems (Weiterstadt). The sequences obtained were aligned and compared with the *TP*53 DNA sequence (accession number x54516) using "BLAST 2 sequences" (http://www.ncbi.nih.gov/gorf/bl2.html). All chromatograms were reviewed manually.

4 RESULTS

4.1 GENE IDENTIFICATION: MICROARRAY HYBRIDISATION

RNA was extracted from 26 tumour samples 10 MPNST, 7 pNFs and 9 dNFs. RNA quality was assessed by RNA agarose gel electrophoresis (Figure 9; A) and checked once more at Scienion with a 2100 bioanalyser by assessing the 28S/18S rRNA ratio (Figure 9; B).

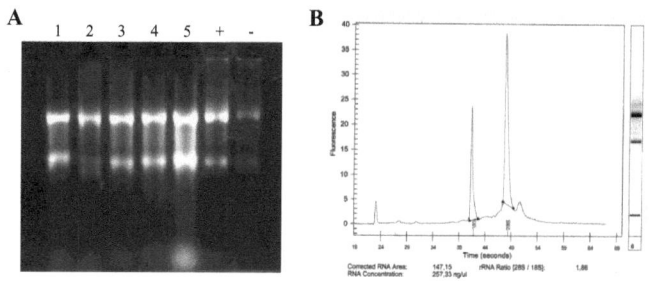

Figure 9: RNA quality verification: RNA quality was checked by agarose gel electrophoresis (1 µg RNAs were loaded) (A) and bioanalyser (B). A good RNA preparation should produce two bands, representing the 28S and the 18S ribosomal RNA subunits (rRNA). The 28S band should be roughly twice as intense as the 18S band. +: positive control; -: negative control (undegraded RNA).

Microarray analysis was performed with the 26 tumour samples and 558 cDNAs. After a strict statistical analysis performed at the Institute of Biochemistry we identified 57 genes showing at least 2-fold expression differences between the 3 tumour entities. The colour coded expression matrix (heat map) of the 57 genes clustered the tumours in 3 groups corresponding to the tumour entities MPNST, pNF and dNF (Figure 10). An exception was the pNF p22476 which clustered within the MPNST group and progressed 2 years later to MPNST M24784. The 2 cell cultures ("z") clustered together in the MPNST group and interestingly showed lower gene expression than the primary tumours. Surprisingly, the cell line M462 did not cluster side by side with MPNST M24472 of which it was cultured

Expression patterns differed gradually from dNFs to pNFs and to MPNST. dNFs and MPNST showed clearly inverse expression patterns. The first 24 genes positioned in the upper part of the heat map discriminate between NFs (pNF and dNF) and MPNST.

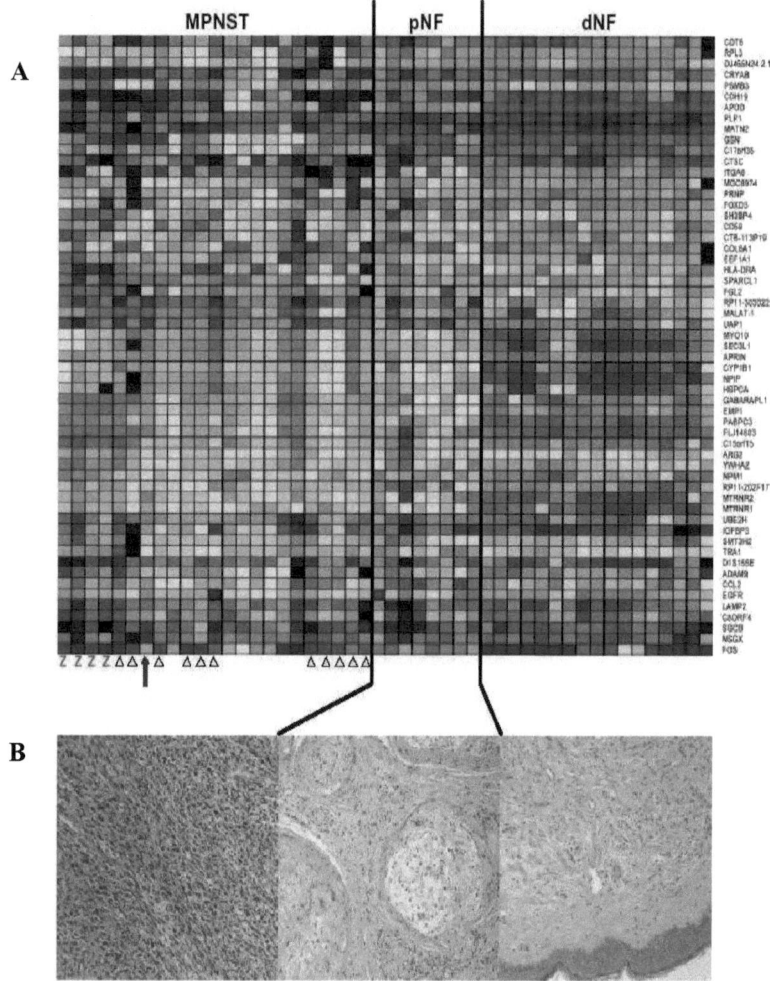

Figure 10: **Heat map and typical histological features of the tumour entities** (N. Holtkamp, 2004): A) High expression levels are represented in red and low expression in blue. Cell lines are indicated with a "z" and sporadic MPNST with a triangle; B) H&E staining with characteristic histologic features for the 3 different tumour types. (ID numbers from left to right: MZ2462a & b, MZ562a & b,M26582a, p22476a, M24784b, M26592a & b, M26596a, M21852a & b,M24472a & b, M21914a & b, M26584a, M26580a & b, M26596b, M26584b, p21410a, p24474a & b, p24994a, p25000b, p24482b, p24996a & b, d25888a & b, d25904b, d25902b, d25898a & b, d25590a, d25894a & b, d25896a &b, 25892a & b, d25900a & b, d259022a)

4.2 VERIFICATION ON THE PROTEIN LEVEL

Microarray analysis was performed to assess differential gene expression. As mRNA level expression does not necessarily correlate with protein levels, it is important to verify the differential gene expression on the protein level to validate their significance in NF1-associated tumourigenesis. Therefore, WBs were performed for matrix metalloproteinase 13 (MMP-13), p53, syndecan-1 and 4 (Syn-1 and Syn-4), platelet derived growth factor receptor alpha (PDGFR-α), prion protein (PrP), proteolipoprotein (PLP), matrilin-2 (mtr-2) and apolipoprotein D (apoD). Furthermore I carried out IF for MMP-13 and IHC for p53, Syn-1 and Syn-4.

4.2.1 MMP-13 EXPRESSION

First, WB for MMP-13 was performed and a unique band of 48 kDa corresponding to the active form of MMP-13 was detected (Figure 11) in 3 MPNST.

Figure 11: **Western blot for MMP-13.** MPNST are printed in red, pNFs in green and dNFs in blue.

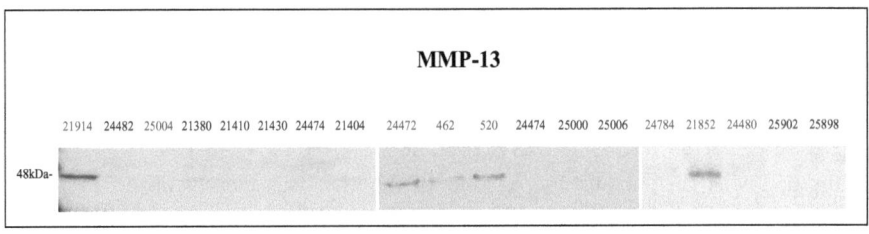

To examine MMP-13 patterns in a larger panel of primary MPNST (n=36) IHC was performed. 5 pNFs and 9 dNFs were also examined. A semiquantitative scoring system was employed to quantify the proportion of stained tumour cells (<5%, -; 5-30%, *; 31-60%, **; >60%, ***). Results are listed in Table 14. Immunocytochemistry was performed for the MPNST cell cultures.

MMP-13 expression was detected in 58% (21/36) of MPNST patients and in both MPNST cell cultures but was absent in the 14 NFs analysed. Cytoplasmatic location of MMP-13 was detected in tumour cells restricted to distinct areas of the tumours (Figure 12). However, 3 MPNST (8%) showed homogeneous MMP-13 distribution, including more than 60% of the cells. The frequency of MMP-13 in sporadic (8/14, 57%) and NF1-associated MPNST (13/22, 59%) was similar.

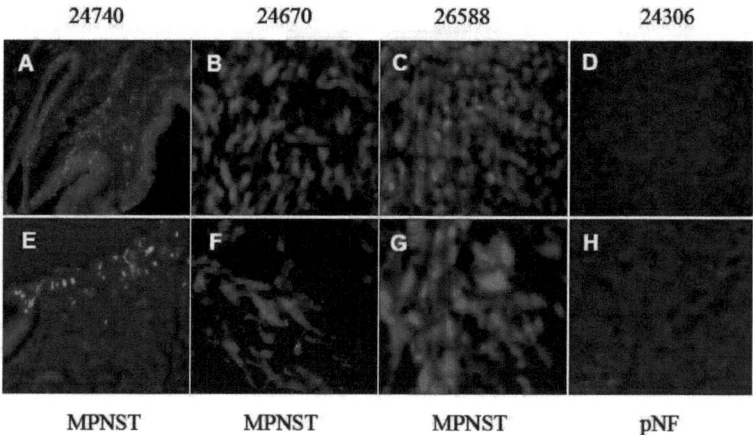

Figure 12: **MMP-13 immunofluorescence**: Representative images of MMP-13 IF staining patterns in 3 MPNST (24740, 24670, 26588) and a pNF (24306). Images A : x100, B-D: x200 magnification; Images E-H: x400 magnification.

4.2.2. P53 Expression

WB for p53 was carried out and a band of 53 kDa was clearly observed for an MPNST and both cell cultures. MPNST 21914 showed a weak signal.

Figure 13: **Western blot for p53.** MPNST are shown in red, pNFs in green and dNFs in blue.

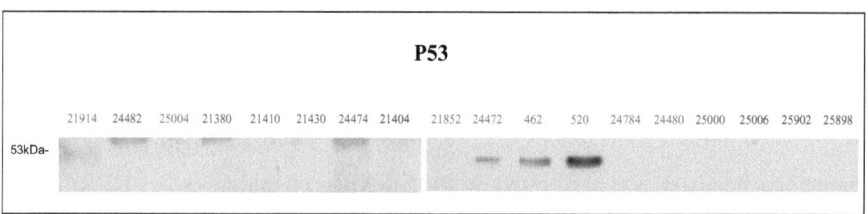

IHC for p53 was performed with 36 MPNST, 5 pNFs, 9 dNFs and both MPNST cell cultures. The following scoring system was used for p53 IHC: 0%, -; 1-5%, +; 6-25%, ++; >25%, +++.

p53 was detected in 78% (28/36) MPNST and in both MPNST cell cultures. NFs lacked p53 staining (Figure 14). Results are listed in Table 14.

Figure 14: p53 IHC: example of an MPNST (24668) with more than 25% of cells positive for p53, an MPNST with 5 to 10% of cells positive for p53 and a pNF negative for p53.

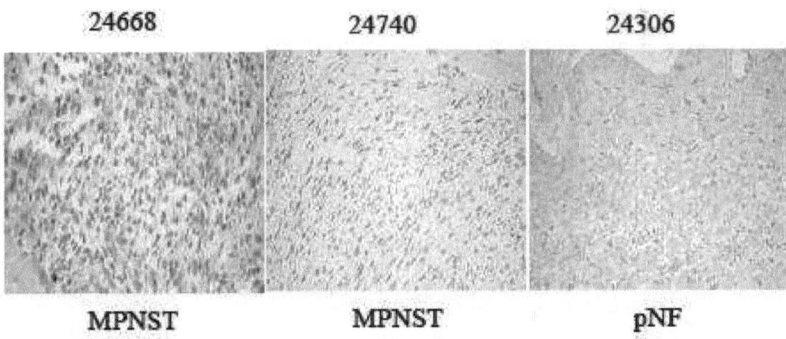

4.2.3 SYNDECANS

Syn-1 and Syn-4 expression in NF1-associated tumours was evaluated by WB and IHC. WB was performed with 3 MPNST, 2 MPNST cell cultures, 6 pNFs and 3 dNFs. IHC for Syn-1 and Syn-4 was studied in 10 MPNST, 9 pNFs and 10 dNFs from 19 different NF1 patients. Slides showing a transition from pNF to MPNST were available from 5 patients.

4.2.3.1 SYNDECAN-1

Syn-1 antibody anti-CD138 proved not to be suitable for WB. Therefore IHC was performed. A semiquantitative scoring system was employed to quantify the proportion of stained tumour cells (<5%, -; 5-30%, +; 31-60%, ++; >60%, +++). Results are listed in Table 11. Syn-1 was found in 90% (9/10) of MPNST and was abundantly expressed in the cytoplasm of cancer cells. In contrast, only 14% of NFs expressed Syn-1. A clear differential expression pattern was observed in tumours with transition of pNF/MPNST. Only the malignant part stained for Syn-1 (Figure 15). The most striking Syn-1 staining was found in poorly differentiated MPNST. It is noteworthy that many of these tumours contained intracellular Syn-1, as evidenced by a perinuclear, granular-type staining pattern (Figure 15; C). Epithelial cell layer, adipocytes as well as occasional plasma cells also stained strongly for Syn-1.

Figure 15: **Syndecan-1 IHC:** Syn-1 staining in 2 MPNST with benign and malignant parts (A-C: 21852; D-F: 24332): the MPNST area is positive for Syn-1 (A, D & F) and the pNF area negative (B & E). Arrow: endothelial cells are not stained by Syn-1. A, B, D and E: x100; C and F: x400 magnification of both MPNST areas showing the granular-type perinuclear staining pattern.

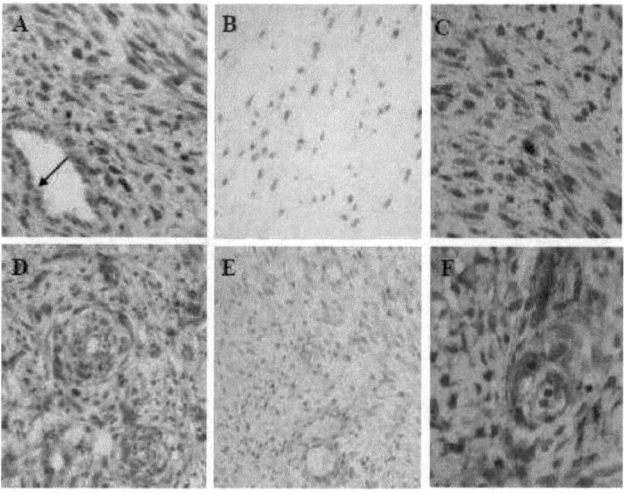

4.2.3.2 SYNDECAN-4

To elucidate the protein expression of Syn-4 in NF1-associated tumours, I performed WB and observed a unique band of approximately 220 kDa. Levels of Syn-4 expression were similar in benign and MPNST. However, Syn-4 expression was slightly increased in NFs.

Figure 16: Syndecan-4 Western blot. MPNST are written in red, pNFs in green and dNFs in blue.

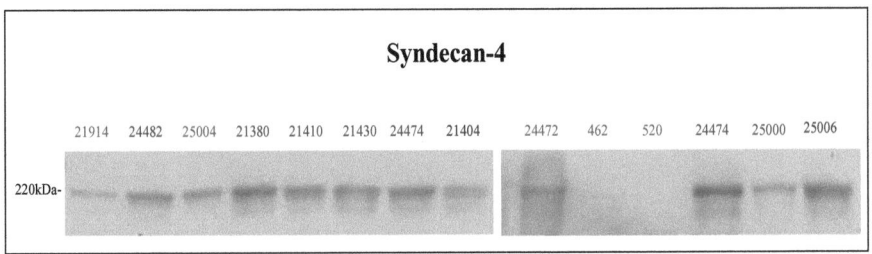

Surprisingly, by IHC only one pNF out of 30 tumours showed tumour cells expressing Syn-4. However, the vascular smooth muscle cells (SMCs) around the blood vessels were strongly stained, as shown in Figure 17, and served as internal control. Although SMCs stained positive for Syn-4 in all NFs, only 46% (7/15) of the MPNST and pNF/MPNST showed SMCs positive Syn-4 staining, usually within the margin of the tumours. Differences in expression patterns were also seen within tumours with transition of pNF/MPNST. Furthermore, NFs showed vessels with increased diameter and intimal hyperplasia.

Figure 17: Syndecan 4 IHC: A-B: dNF (21908) Tumour cells did not express Syn-4 in contrast to the cells of the basal layer of the epidermis that served as internal control; C-D pNF (24192): this tumour was the only one of 30 showing Syn-4 expression in tumour cells; E and F: Comparison of the blood vessels in a pNF (24324) and a MPNST (21852), respectively: in both tumours Syn-4 was not expressed by tumour cells, however SMCs stained positive in NFs (Figure C). Furthermore, blood vessels had an increased diameter in pNFs than in MPNST. Intimal hyperplasia was observed in NFs. Arrows show blood vessels.

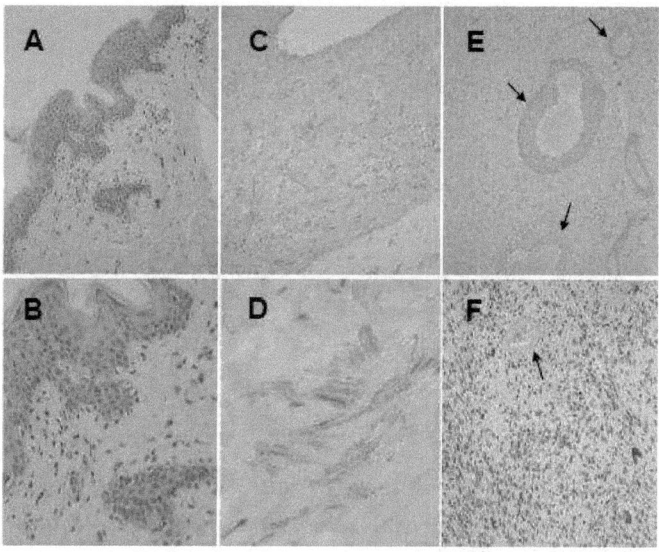

Table 11: Results of Syn-1 and Syn-4 IHC in dNFs, pNFs and MPNST; T: tumour cells; V: blood vessels; Out: within the margin of the tumour.

	ID-Number	Tumour type	Localisation	Syndecan-1	Syndecan-4
1	24356	dNF	Unknown	-	T-; V+
2	24358	dNF	Unknown	-	T-; V+
3	24338	dNF	Leg distal	-	T-; V+
4	24350	dNF	Leg distal	-	T-; V+
5	24328	dNF	Unknown	-	NP
6	24294	dNF	Thoracic wall	-	T-; V+
7	22464	dNF	Cheek	-	T-; V+
8	22460	dNF	Thoracic wall	+	T-; V+
9	21908	dNF	Unknown	-	T-; V+
10	21402	dNF	Unknown	-	T-; V+
11	21380	pNF	Cheek	+	T-; V+
12	24192	pNF	Unknown	-	T++; V+
13	24222	pNF	Skin	-	T-; V+ out
14	24306	pNF	N. ischiadicus	-	T-; V+ out
15	21852	pNF/MPNST	Intra- und extraspinal	+++	T-;V-/ T-; V-
16	24324	pNF/MPNST	Leg	+	T-;V+/T-; V+
17	24332	pNF/MPNST	Arm distal	++	T-;V+/ T-;V-
18	24334	pNF/MPNST	Unknown	-	T-;V+/ T-;V-
19	24354	pNF/MPNST	Unknown	-	T-;V+/ T-;V-
20	21914	MPNST	Leg proximal	++	T-; V-
21	22318	MPNST	Sacro	+	T-; V-
22	22568	MPNST	Intraspinal	+++	T-; V-
23	24256	MPNST	Arm distal	+++	T-; V-
24	24308	MPNST	Leg proximal	-	T-; V-
25	24314	MPNST	Thoracic wall	+++	T-; V+
26	24316	MPNST	Thoracic wall	++	T-; V+ out
27	24322	MPNST	Plexus cervicobrachialis	+++	T-; V-
28	24326	MPNST	Plexus cervicobrachialis	+++	T-; V-
29	24694	MPNST	Leg distal	+++	T-; V+ out

4.2.4 PLATELET-DERIVED GROWTH FACTOR RECEPTOR ALPHA

Differential expression of PDGFR-α was first identified by SSH and confirmed by virtual Northern blotting (vNB) to be 15-fold higher in MPNST. WB Was performed to validate the previous results. A unique band of approximately 185 kDa was observed in MPNST and a thinner band in some NFs, corresponding to PDGFR-α (Figure 18).

Figure 18: Western blot for PDGFR-α. MPNST are shown in red, pNFs in green and dNFs in blue.

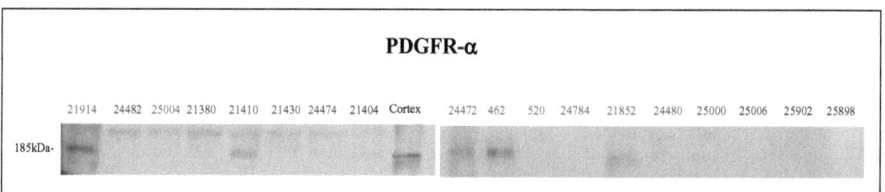

4.2.5 PRION PROTEIN

PrP mRNA was identified to be more strongly expressed in pNFs than in MPNST by SSH and confirmed by vNB. By WB I observed 3 bands of approximately 27, 30 and 37 kDa, corresponding to the non-, mono- and diglycosylated forms of PrP. NFs showed stronger expression levels of PrP than MPNST and was most commonly monoglycosylated. As positive controls, cortex lysates, which showed high expression of PrP, were utilised.

Figure 19: Western blot for prion protein. MPNST are written in red, pNFs in green and dNFs inblue.

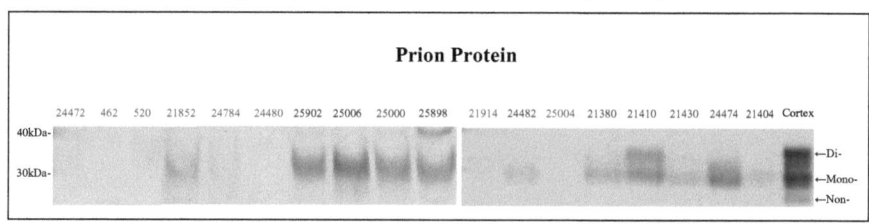

4.2.6 PROTEOLIPID PROTEIN

PLP was first identified by SSH and confirmed by vNB to be overexpressed in NFs[74]. Furthermore, microarray analysis validated these results and confirmed the overexpression of PLP mRNA in NFs[75]. By WB I observed 2 bands of 26 and 20.5 kDa corresponding to the *PLP* gene products PLP (26 kDa) and DM-20 (20.5 kDa). Although DM-20 levels were similar in all tumour types, PLP was only present in MPNST, especially in both MPNST cell cultures.

Figure 20: Western blot for proteolipid protein. MPNST are written in red, pNFs in green and dNFs in blue.

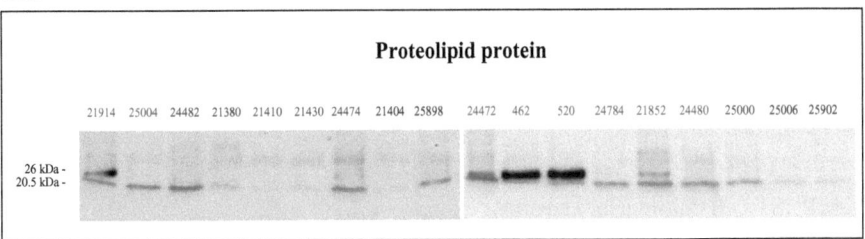

4.2.7 MATRILIN-2

In previous studies mtr-2 mRNA was observed to be differentially expressed in NF1-associated tumours by SSH, vNB and microarray analysis[74, 75]. To elucidate mtr-2 protein expression in NF1-associated tumours, I performed WB.

Figure 21: Western blot for matrilin-2. MPNST are written in red, pNFs in green and dNFs in blue.

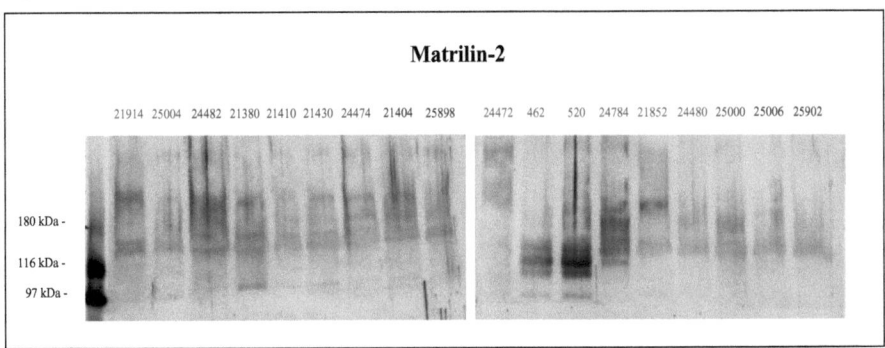

Both MPNST cell cultures and a MPNST showed a band of the expected molecular mass (≈125 kDa) for the mtr-2 polypeptide, plus a smaller band (≈ 100 kDa), probably representing a proteolytic breakdown product. However, mtr-2 was not expressed among the rest of NF1-associated tumours. The oligomers of different sizes we observed likely represent modified products or unspecific bands due to the usage of an unpurified serum.

4.2.8 APOLIPOPROTEIN D

ApoD mRNA was found to be overexpressed in NFs by SSH and microarray analysis. I next examined apoD protein expression in NF1-associated tumours by WB. A band of ≈29 kDa was observed in all tumour types examined. However, lower levels of apoD were detected in primary MPNST in comparison to NFs. Furthermore, both MPNST cell cultures lacked apoD expression.

Figure 22: **Western blot for Apolipoprotein D.** MPNST are written in red, pNFs in green and dNfs in blue.

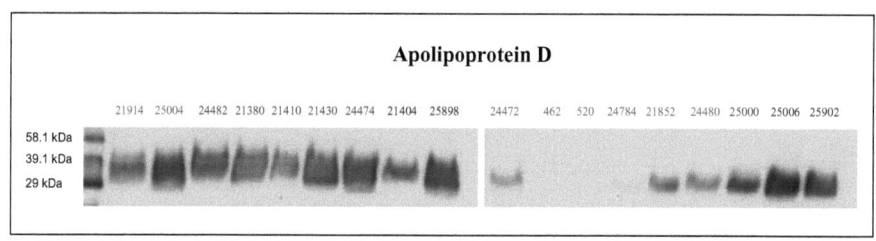

All WB results are summarised in Table 12.

Table 12: WB results for MMP-13, p53, Syn-4, PDGFR-α, PrP, PLP, Mtr-2 and ApoD. NP: not performed

ID	Tumour	MMP-13	P53	Syn-4	PDGFR-α	PrP	PLP	Mtr-2	ApoD
21914	MPNST	+	+	+	++	-	+	-	++
25004	MPNST	-	-	++	-	-	-	-	++
24742	MPNST	+	+	++	+	-	+	-	+
24784	MPNST	-	-	NP	-	-	-	-	+
21852	MPNST	+	-	NP	++	+	+	+	+
24880	MPNST	-	-	NP	-	-	-	-	+
462	MPNST	+	+	-	+	-	++	++	-
520	MPNST	+	+	-	-	-	++	++	-
24882	pNF	-	-	++	-	+	-	-	++
21380	pNF	-	-	++	-	+	-	-	++
21410	pNF	-	-	++	+	++	-	-	++
21430	pNF	-	-	++	-	+	-	-	++
24774	pNF	-	-	++	-	++	-	-	++
25000	pNF	-	-	+	-	++	-	-	++
21404	dNF	-	-	+	+	+	-	-	++
25006	dNF	-	-	++	-	++	-	-	++
25902	dNF	-	-	++	-	++	-	-	++
25898	dNF	-	-	++	-	++	-	-	++

4.3 MMP-13 AND P53

4.3.1 IS MMP13 EXPRESSION INDUCED BY MUTANT P53?

P53 has been shown to regulate the promoter activity of invasion-associated proteinases such as MMP-1, MMP-2 and MMP-13[76]. Wild-type p53 repressed MMP-13 promotor, however some p53 mutants were found to lose their inhibitory effect or even to stimulate MMP13 expression up to 2-3 fold[76].

MMP-13 expression was observed in 58% of MPNST and p53 in 78% of MPNST. It is worthy of note that a highly significant association between MPNST expression p53- and MMP-13 was found (p=0.005; Fisher exact test). Taking into account the different staining levels, the association was still significant (p=0.02; Pearson correlation). To find out whether mutant p53 was responsible for MMP-13 expression in vivo, a panel of 36 MPNST was screened for *TP53* mutations. The entire coding and promoter region (exon 1 to 11) was checked for *TP53* sequence alterations.

Somatic mutations were detected in 4 of 36 MPNST (11%) and in both MPNST cell cultures within the exons 4, 5, 7 and 9. MPNST 24256 carried a mutation that results in a stop codon at position 321 (AAA>TAA). The NF1-associated MPNST 24472 and the corresponding cell culture S462 carried a mutation in codon 110 (CGT>CCT; Arg>Pro). Both MPNST belonged to NF1 patients. Two *TP53* mutations were detected in sporadic MPNST. MPNST 26582 carried a mutation in codon 258 (GAA>GCA; Glu>Ala) and MPNST 26588 in codon 173 (GTG>ATG; Val>Met).

TP53 mutation analysis

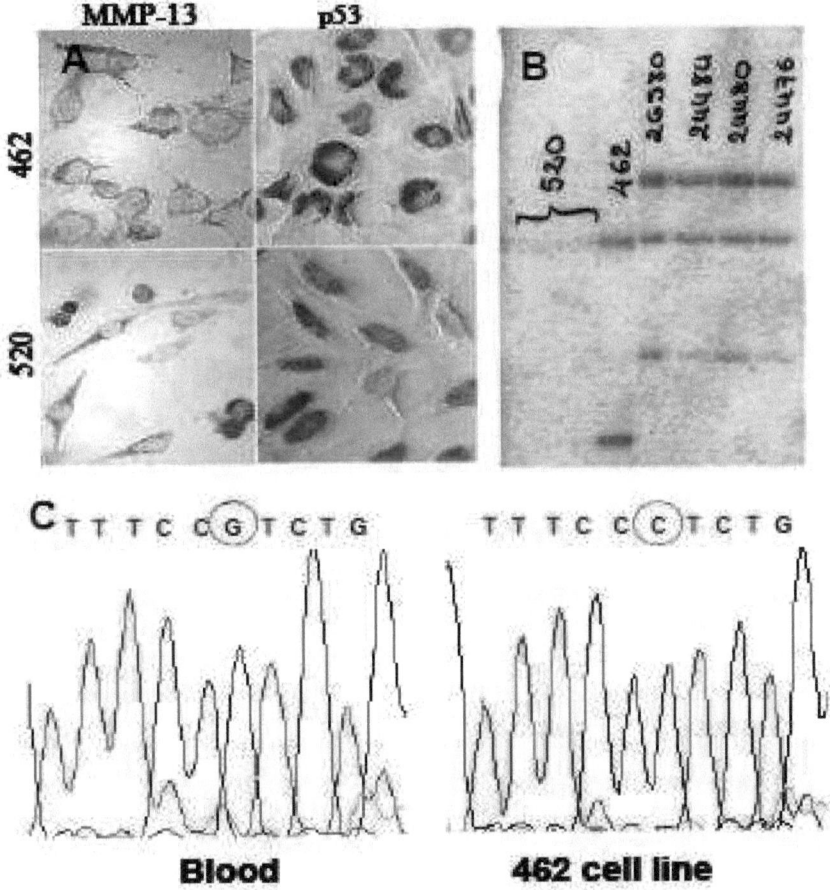

Figure 23: *TP53* **mutation analysis and MMP-13 and p53 immunocytochemistry** A) Cytochemistry showing localisation of MMP-13 and p53 staining in 462 and 520 MPNST cell cultures. B) SSCP analysis showing a different running behaviour for PCR products of 462 and 520 MPNST cell cultures C) A mutation in exon 4, codon 110, CGT>CCT, was evidenced by sequencing in the MPNST cell culture 462.

Figure 24: Distribution of the most common *TP53* mutation sites in tumours. Most *TP53* mutations are missense mutations in the DNA binding domain. The localisation of the mutations observed in our study are marked with a ▲. Modified picture from: www-p53.iarc.fr

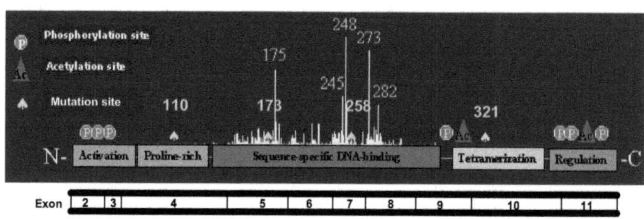

MPNST harboring a *TP53* mutation were associated with higher amounts of p53 immunopositive cells (p=0.017; Pearson correlation). However, *TP53* mutations were not significantly associated with MMP-13 expression (p=0.141; Fisher exact test).

Four different polymorphisms in intron 2, intron 3 and exon 4 of *TP53* were detected (Table 13). The silent polymorphism in exon 6 (codon 213, A>G) was not detected. Thirteen patients were heterozygous and one was homozygous for the C^{11827} allele in intron 2. The allele frequency was $f(C^{11827}= 0.21)$. Eleven patients were heterozygous for the 16bp duplication in intron 3 $f(dup^{16bp}=0.15)$ and 3 patients were heterozygous for the A^{11992} allele corresponding to $f(A^{11992}= 0.041)$. Fifteen patients were heterozygous for the p53Pro^{72} allele corresponding to $f(Pro^{72}= 0.21)$ and $f(Arg^{72}= 0.79)$. To exactly determine allele frequency of the exon 4 polymorphism we determined blood DNA in addition to tumor DNA, which might contain allelic loss. Loss of heterozygosity was found in MPNST 24256. Allele frequencies were compared to control groups published in previous studies[77, 78]. No significant differences were observed.

Table 13: *TP53* polymorphisms in MPNST patients. Position of polymorphisms are given according to reference X54156 from GenBank. na: nucleic acid; f: allele frequency

Localisation		DNA alteration	N° of cases	f MPNST patients	f controls
Intron 2	na 11827	G to C	13 heterozygous 1 homozygous	C^{11827} 0.21	C^{11827} 0.31
Intron 3	na 11951	Duplication GGGGA-CCTGGAGGCT	11 heterozygous	16bp dup 0.15	16bp dup 0.16
Intron 3	na 11992	C to A	3 heterozygous	A^{11992} 0.032	A^{11992} 0.041
Exon 4	codon 72	CGC>CCC	15 heterozygous	$p53Pro^{72}$ 0.21	$p53Pro^{72}$ 0.26

4.3.2 RELEVANCE OF MMP-13 EXPRESSION AND *TP53* STATUS IN MPNST PATIENTS

4.3.2.1 CLINICAL DESCRIPTION OF THE MPNST PATIENTS

The study contained MPNST from 36 patients. Only tumours from patients with complete clinical information were taken for statistical analysis. Information on patients and tumours is provided in Table 14. Twenty-two patients were diagnosed with NF1 while 14 patients developed sporadic MPNST. The female/male ratio in both groups was 1:1. The mean age at tumour diagnosis was 32.6 years for patients with NF1 and 52.4 years for patients with sporadic MPNST and differed significantly (T-test; p=0.003). The mean time of follow-up was 40.56 months, 49.2 months for NF1 patients and 27.1 months for sporadic MPNST (p=0.214, T-test). Twenty-two tumours located axially and 14 in the periphery. Patient with peripheral tumour location had a better

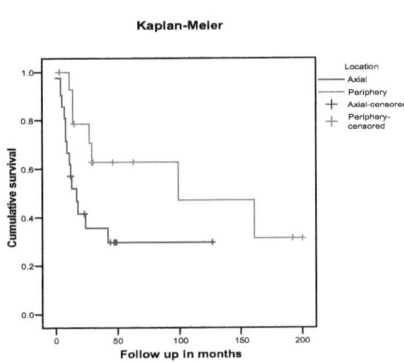

Figure 25: Survival of MPNST patients depending on tumour location

prognosis as shown on survival analysis (p=0.045; log rank, p=0.022; Breslow) compared with axial tumour location (Figure 25). Local recurrence occurred in 44.4% (16/36) of patients, 54.5% (12/22) in NF1 patients and 33.3% (4/12) in sporadic MPNST (p=0.176, Fischer exact test), after a mean interval of 18.1 months, 21.5 months for NF1 patients and 8 months for sporadic MPNST (p=0.499, T-test). The tumour metastasised in 14 of 36 (38.9%) patients, 31.8% (7/22) of NF1 patient and 50% (7/14) of sporadic MPNST (p=0.275, Π^2) after a mean interval of 13 months, 20.9 for NF1 patients and 5.1 months for sporadic MPNST (p=0.421, T-test). Tumour dissemination was most frequently to the lung (78.6%). No differences on cumulative survival between both NF1-associated and sporadic MPNST was observed (p= 0.774; log rank). The 5 year-survival rate was 16.7%, 18.2% for NF1 patients and 16.7% for sporadic MPNST patients. Survival analysis did not show any gender difference (p=0.998; log rank).

4.3.2.2 CLINICAL RELEVANCE OF MMP-13 EXPRESSION AND *TP53* STATUS IN MPNST PATIENTS

MMP-13 expression in MPNST was significantly associated with relapse (p=0.019; Fisher exact test). This association was even stronger when taking into account the different staining levels (p=0.013; Fisher exact test). In detail, only 20% MPNST negative for MMP-13 relapsed. In contrast, increasing levels of MMP-13 expression increase the proportion of patient with relapse (+: 46% MPNST patients relapsed; ++: 80%

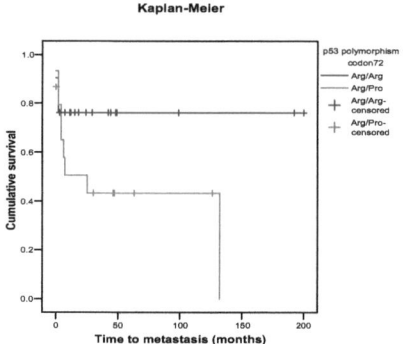

Figure 26: Time to occurrence of metastasis in MPNST patients carrying the *TP53* Pro[72] allele

MPNST patient relapsed; +++: 100% MPNST patient relapsed). Cumulative survival analysis, however, was of borderline significance (p=0.055; log rank).

TP53 mutations were not significantly associated with MMP-13 expression (p=0.141; Fisher exact test) but with histological grade (p=0.020; Pearson correlation). All MPNST with mutant *TP53* were histological grade 3. Metastatic disease was associated with the p53Pro^{72} polymorphism (p=0.028; Π^2) and correlated with shorter survival (p=0.0007; log rank) (Figure 26). No significant association was detected for MMP-13 expression with p53Pro^{72} polymorphism. Furthermore, MMP-13 was not linked to metastasis.

Results

Table 14: Patient and tumour characteristics. ID: tumour identification number. NF1: NF1 status of the patient. †: dead patient. Grade: tumour grade according to the modified FNCLCC system. IF: immunofluorescence. IHC: immunohistochemistry. p53 mut: p53 mutation status. p53 pol.: p53 polymorphism. N: C^{11992}. Dup: 16bp duplication. Lower part of the table contains non-NF1 patients.

ID	Sex/Age	NF1	Follow up month	Localisation	Grade	Metastasis localisation/month	Relapse month	MMP-13 IF	P53 IHC	p53 mut	P53 pol. codon 72	TP53 pol. Intron 2	TP53 pol. Intron 3
21852	M/29	Yes	24†	Intraspinal	2	-	6	+	+	-	Arg/Arg	G/G	N/N
24256	F/21	Yes	161†	Arm distal	3	Lungs, liver, pancreas, lymph nodes/132	108	++	++	p53 nonsense	Arg/Pro	C/LOH	Dup/LOH
24320	M/56	Yes	46	leg	1	-	-	+	++	-	Arg/Pro	C/G	Dup/N
24626	M/58	Yes	49	Back	2	-	-	+	++	-	Arg/Arg	G/G	N/N
24472	F/19	Yes	11†	Leg proximal	3	-	2	+	++	p53 Pro 116	Arg/Arg	G/G	N/N
21914	F/21	Yes	30	Leg proximal	2	-	4	+	+	-	Arg/Arg	G/G	Dup/N
24304	M/27	Yes	17†	Plexus cervicobrachialis	1	Paravertebral, lumbal, thoracic/0	14	++	+	-	Arg/Arg	G/G	N/N
24308	M/21	Yes	14†	Leg proximal	3	Lung, thoracic wall/6	-	+	+++	-	Arg/Pro	C/G	Dup/N
24310	M/66	Yes	8†	trunk	2	Lung/2	5	-	-	-	Arg/Pro	C/G	N/N
24326	M/52	Yes	8†	Plexus cervicobrachialis	2	Lung/2	-	-	+	-	Arg/Arg	G/G	N/N
24332	F/30	Yes	192	Arm distal	2	-	10	++	++	-	Arg/Arg	G/G	Dup/N
24354	F/33	Yes	200	Leg distal	1	-	96	+	++	-	Arg/Arg	G/G	N/N
24476	F/13	Yes	99†	Arm distal	2	-	-	-	-	-	Arg/Arg	G/G	N/N
24480	F/20	Yes	71	Mediastino	2	-	-	-	-	-	Arg/Arg	G/G	N/N
24484	F/31	Yes	18†	Gluteo	3	-	4	-	++	-	Arg/Arg	G/G	Dup/N
24534	F/28	Yes	44	Thoracic wall	3	-	-	-	+++	-	Arg/Arg	G/G	Dup/N
24668	F/14	Yes	9†	Intraspinal	3	Lung/0	3	+++	++	-	Arg/Arg	C/C	Dup/N
24670	M/31	Yes	13†	Inspinal	3	Lung/4	4	-	+	-	Arg/Pro	C/G	A11992/N
24694	F/79	Yes	29	Leg distal	2	-	-	+	++	-	Arg/Arg	G/G	N/N
24748	M/34	Yes	12†	Gluteo	2	-	2	++	++	-	Arg/Arg	C/G	N/N
24772	M/15	Yes	42†	Retroperitoneal	2	-	-	-	+	-	Arg/Arg	C/G	N/N
24776	M/39	Yes	48	right axilla	1	-	-	++	+	-	Arg/Arg	G/G	N/N
26580	F/78	No	41	Gluteo	3	Lung/0	-	-	++	p53 Ala 28	Arg/Arg	G/G	A11992/N
26582	M/43	No	126	Os ileum	3	-	-	+	++	-	Arg/Pro	C/G	N/N
26584	M/41	No	47	Plexus cervicobrachialis	2	-	-	-	-	-	Arg/Pro	G/G	N/N
26586	M/28	No	27†	Leg distal	2	Lung/0	-	+	+	-	Arg/Arg	G/G	N/N
26588	F/73	No	63	Leg proximal	3	-	-	+++	+++	p53 Met 175	Arg/Pro	C/G	Dup/N
26590	F/50	No	11†	Gluteo	2	Lung/0	-	-	-	-	Arg/Arg	G/G	N/N
26592	F/72	No	0†	Liver	2	-	-	+	+	-	Arg/Pro	G/G	A11992/N
26594	F/55	No	29†	Leg proximal	3	Retroperitoneal/25	-	+	-	-	Arg/Pro	G/G	N/N
28650	F/16	No	12	Intraspinal lumbal	2	-	12	+	-	-	Ara/Ara	G/G	N/N
27772	M/69	No	3	Leg proximal	3	-	3	+	+++	-	Ara/Ara	G/G	N/N
28652	M/73	No	15	Arm distal	1	-	15	++	-	-	Ara/Ara	G/G	N/N
27724	M/47	No	11†	Leg proximal	3	Lung/7	-	+	+	-	Arg/Pro	G/G	Dup/N
30342	F/14	No	51	Intraspinal	2	Shin/4	2	+++	+	-	Arg/Pro	G/G	Dup/N
27752	M/55	No	23	Gluteo	3	Lung/0	-	-	-	-	Arg/Pro	G/G	N/N

5 DISCUSSION

5.1 GENE IDENTIFICATION: MICROARRAY ANALYSIS

Microarray analysis is a screening method performed in order to identify differential gene expression. As NF1 patients develop dNFs, pNFs and MPNST, they provide a perfect system to study the expression of genes involved in the different steps of tumourigenesis.

Evaluation of the gene array data led to the identification of 57 genes, 43 of which were identified for the first time while 14 genes had already been identified by SSH. Hierarchical clustering clearly separated the samples into three groups: dNF, pNF and MPNST. Comparison of expression profiles in NF1-associated and sporadic MPNST did not show any significant difference and suggests related molecular mechanisms of pathogenesis.

Among the genes overexpressed in MPNST, some candidates have already been described in other malignancies. *ADAM9* was found to be upregulated in pancreatic ductal adenocarcinomas and associated with poor tumour differentiation and shorter overall survival[79]. Arginase 2 (*ARG2*) was shown to be overexpressed in follicular thyroid carcinoma[80]. *CYP1B1*, overexpressed in a range of human malignancies[81, 82], can activate a variety of human carcinogens and inactivate the anticancer drug paclitaxel[83]. *MALAT-1*, a non-coding RNA, was first identified to be significantly associated with metastasis in non-small cell lung cancer patients[84]. Myosin X (*MYO10*) overexpression causes an increase in the number and length of filopodia and could be involved in tumour cell invasion[85, 86]. Another interesting point is the overexpression of nucleophosmin (*NPM1*), a natural repressor of p53, able to inhibit p53 transcriptional activity by more than 70% in response to UV light.

Discussion

Overexpression of *NPM1* could contribute to p53 inactivation and tumour progression[87]. Epidermal growth factor receptor (*EGFR*) is overexpressed and/or constitutively activated in a variety of human malignancies and is associated with decreased survival. It is noteworthy that *EGFR* overexpression has been identified as an early event in NF1-associated tumourigenesis. *EGFR* receptor antagonists are already undergoing clinical trials[88-91] and gefitinib is already approved for lung cancer treatment.

Table 15: List including the 57 genes identified to be differentially expressed with detailed sequence annotation and accession number, as well as main function (SMP: Signal and membrane protein; NP: Nuclear protein; ECP: Extracellular protein; FPP: Folding and/or processing protein; MP: metabolic protein; CP: Cytoskeletal protein; OP: Other protein; UP: Unknown function). The genes previously identified by SSH are marked in blue (bold). # marks genes best suited for differentiating between dNFs and pNFs.

Gene symbol	Gene name	Accession	Function
CDT6	Angiopoietin-like factor	XM_00152	ECP
RPL3	Ribosomal protein L3	NM_00096	NP
DJ465N24.2.1	hypothetical protein DJ465N24.2.1	XM_04476	UP
CRYAB	Crystalline alpha B	NM_00188	FPP
PSMB3	Proteasome subunit, beta type 3	BC013008	MP
CDH19	Cadherin 19, type 2	NM_02115	SMP
APOD	Apolipoprotein D	NM_00164	ECP
PLP1	Proteolipid protein	M27110	ECP
MTR-2	Matrilin 2	NM_00021	ECP
GSN	Gelsolin	XM016545	CP
C17orf35	putative receptor protein	XM_04270	UP
CTSC	Cathepsin C, transcript variant 1	NM_00181	OP
ITGA6	Integrin alpha 6	NM_00021	SMP
MGC8974	Hypothetical protein MGC8974	BC013101	UP
PRNP	Prion protein	M13899	SMP
FOXD3	Forkheadbox D3	NM_01218	UP
SH3BP4	SH3-domain binding protein 4	NM_01452	UP
CD59	CD59 antigen p18-20	BC001506	SMP
CTB-113P19	CTB-113P19	AC011374	UP
COL6A1	Collagen, type VI, alpha 1	XM_03620	ECP
EEF1A1	Elongation factor 1 alpha subunit	X03558	NP
HLA-DRA	HLA-DR alpha	NM_01911	SMP

SPARCL1		Hevin	NM_00468	ECP
FGL2		Fibrinogen-like 2	AF468959	ECP
RP11-303O22		RP11-303O22	AC119034	UP
MALAT-1	#	metastasis-associated in lung adenocarcinoma	AF203815	OP
UAP-1	#	UDP-N-acetylglucosamine	BC009377	MP
MYO10	#	Myosin X	NM_01233	CP
SEC3L1	#	Sec3-like	NM_01826	OP
APRIN	#	Androgen-induced proliferation inhibitor	XM_01657	OP
CYP1B1	#	Cytochrome P450 subfamily I	XM_00257	MP
NPIP	#	Nuclear pore complex interacting protein	XM_05373	NP
HSPCA	#	Heat shock protein 90 alpha-like 1	D87666	FPP
GABARAPL1	#	GABA(A) receptor-associated protein-like 1	NM_03141	SMP
EMP1	#	Epithelial membrane protein 1	XM_00688	SMP
PABPC3	#	Poly (A) binding protein, cytoplasmatic 3	BC041863	MP
FLJ14803	#	FLJ14803	NM_03284	UP
C15orf15		60S ribosomal protein L30 isolog	AF201949	NP
ARG2		Arginase, type II	NM_00117	OP
YWHAZ		14-3-3 zeta/Phospholipase A2	M86400	MP
NPM1		Nucleophosmin	BC050628	NP
RP11-202F17		RP11-202F17	AC091808	UP
MTRNR2		16s ribosomal RNA	NC_001807	NP
MTRNR1	#	12s ribosomal RNA	AY012236	NP
UBE2H		Ubiquitin conjugating enzymeUbcH2	Z29331	FPP
IGFBP3		Insulin-like growth factor binding prot. 3	M31159	ECP
SMT3H2		SMT3 suppressor of mif two 3 homolog 2	BC062713	UP
TRA1		Tumour rejection antigen 1	NM_00329	FPP
D1S155E		NRAS-related gene	BC032446	SMP
ADAM9		Disintegrin	NM_00381	ECP
CCL2		Monocyte chemoattractant protein	S69738	ECP
EGFR		Epidermal growth factor receptor	NM_00522	SMP
LAMP2		Lysosome-associated membrane protein-2	X77196	OP
C8ORF4		Open reading frame 4	XM_00526	UP
SGCP		Sarcoglycan β	Y09781	OP
NSGX	#	Brain and nasopharyngeal carcinoma	NM_01441	UP
FOS	#	Fos protooncogen	K00650	NP

Heat shock protein 90 alpha-like 1 (*HSPCA*) is also overexpressed in many solid tumours. Interestingly, *HSPCA* target proteins include several proteins involved in cancer progression such as wild-type and mutant *AR*, wild-type or mutant *KIT*, *ERBB2*, and *AKT1*. The targeting of *HSPCA* is emerging as a potential strategy for cancer treatment. Identification of target genes for developing new therapeutic strategies is of great importance due to the dismal prognosis of the patients affected by MPNST and the lack, currently, of successful therapy. Among the genes overexpressed in NFs (both dNF and pNF), *CDT6*, *APOD*, *PLP1* and *MTR-2* are of special interest. They have been previously identified by SSH[74]. *CDT6*, an angiopoietin-like factor highly expressed in cornea, is thought to block the angiopoietin receptor contributing to cornea avascularity[92]. Therefore, lack of *CDT6* expression in MPNST may contribute to the high vascularity of these tumours. Apoliprotein D (*APOD*), an androgen-regulated hydrophobic transported protein, was identified as a marker for low grade primary CNS neoplasms[93]. Lack of *APOD* expression was a predictor of shorter survival in patients with non-resectable prostate cancer[94]. Proteolipid protein *PL(P)*, as well as *EMP1*, encode components of the myelin sheath. *PLP* are involved in maintenance of the myelin sheath in the PNS[95, 96]. Overexpression of *EMP1* inhibits growth of the esophageal squamous carcinoma cell line EC9706 and arrests the cells in S phase. Matrilin-2 (*MTRNR2*) and collagen 6 (*COL6A1*) are ECM proteins. Their overexpression in NFs corresponds to the higher quantity of ECM in NFs than in MPNST. Moreover, proteins involved in cell-cell adhesion or interaction with the ECM such as *CDH19* and *ITGA6* were also highly expressed in NFs.

DNFs and pNFs are benign tumours, however 30% of pNFs progress to MPNST. Therefore, it would be important to find markers able to distinguish between borderline tumours. By microarray analysis, we identified 15 genes that discriminate between pNFs and dNFs (labelled with # in Table 12). *FOS*, up regulated in pNFs but not in dNFs and MPNST, could be used in clinic as a diagnostic marker to discriminate borderline tumours. Interestingly, *FOS* expression was first identified by SSH and confirmed by vNB to show 100-fold higher expression in pNFs than in MPNST[74]. An independent study showed that *FOS* was among the most discriminatory genes able to distinguish between pNFs and MPNST[64]. *FOS* expression in pNFs was more than 14 times stronger than in MPNST.

In conclusion, microarray analysis provides a catalogue of interesting genes that contributes to a better understanding of the mechanisms involved in NF1-tumourigenesis. The identification of genes that may serve as diagnostic, prognostic or therapeutic markers will allow patients to receive an individual management, obtaining the optimal treatment for their pathology.

5.2 VERIFICATION ON THE PROTEIN LEVEL

The expression of genetic information in all cells is a one way system: DNA→RNA→protein. This constitutes the central dogma of molecular biology. DNA specifies the synthesis of RNA and RNA the synthesis of polypeptides, which subsequently form proteins. However, only a small proportion of genes in cells are transcribed, according to the needs of the cell. Moreover, only a portion of the RNA is translated to polypeptides. The steady-state rate of a given mRNA depends on the balance between its rates of synthesis and degradation. mRNA levels are modulated through transcriptional and posttranscriptional mechanisms such as RNA splicing, capping and polyadenylation. In addition, mRNA surveillance pathways prevent the synthesis of truncated proteins, which can have dominant-negative and other deleterious effects. Another important posttranscriptional control is exerted by mRNA stability through cis-acting elements such as AREs (AU rich elements) and trans-acting factors. AREs are defined by their ability to promote rapid mRNA decay[97]. Furthermore, the destabilizing activity of AREs can be increased or decreased as a result of interactions with AUBPs (AU binding proteins).

Both SSH and microarray analysis were performed to assess differential gene expression on the mRNA level. As mRNA translation can be modulated, it is important to verify if the differential expression is also observed on the protein level. Therefore, we performed WB, IHC and/or IF.

5.2.1 MMP13 AND P53

5.2.1.1 MMP13

Invasion of surrounding tissues by neoplastic cells is one of the most important steps in tumour progression. Matrix metalloproteinases (MMPs) are a 26-member family of zinc-dependent endopeptidases, capable of degrading most ECM components. Secreted as latent precursor (zymogen), MMP-13 is proteolytic activated in the extracellular space. Notably, MMP-13 is able to degrade a wide spectrum of ECM components, including type II, IV, X, XIV collagens, fibronectin, tenascin and fibrillin[98-100]. MMP-13 plays an important role in physiological conditions such as wound healing and embryogenesis[101] as well as in pathological situations such as atherosclerosis, rheumatoid arthritis, tumour invasion, metastasis and tumour angiogenesis[102-105].

MMP-13 was initially identified to be overexpressed in breast cancer[106] and later in several other malignant tumours, including chondrosarcoma[107], head and neck carcinomas[108, 109], basal cell carcinoma[110], malignant melanoma[111] and vulvar carcinoma[102]. Furthermore, these studies revealed that MMP-13 expression associates with invasive and metastatic features, supporting the idea that MMP-13 can serve as a prognostic marker. As invasion of cancer cells is a multistep process that involves enhanced cellular motility and proteolytic activity, it has been suggested that MMP-13 plays an important role in invasion and metastasis.

MMP-13 was first identified by SSH to be more strongly expressed in MPNST than in NFs[74]. Recently, MMP-13 was observed by RT-PCR to be strongly overexpressed in MPNST in comparison to pNFs[112]. In the present study, we showed that the active form of MMP-13 is expressed by tumour cells in 58% of MPNST as well as by 2 MPNST cell cultures. MMP-13 expression was similar in NF1-associated and sporadic MPNST. In contrast, MMP-13 was not observed in pNFs or in dNFs. Because MPNST usually develop from pre-existent pNFs the gain of MMP-13 expression indicates a role for MMP-13 in malignant transformation. In this study, MMP-13 expression was confined to tumour cells which show quite a variable and heterogeneous expression pattern, usually restricted to the invasive margin of the tumour. It is noteworthy that MMP-13 is one of the few MMPs specifically expressed by tumour cells in malignant tumours, whereas most MMPs are expressed by stromal fibroblasts or tumour infiltrating inflammatory cells[113].

5.2.1.2 P53

p53 is a transcription factor involved in cell cycle control, DNA repair and apoptosis. Because of its physiological role in the maintenance of genomic stability, p53 has also been designated the guardian of the genome.

In our panel of 36 MPNST, p53 immunostaining was detected in 78% of MPNST and in both MPNST cell cultures. All NFs lacked p53 staining. Due to the short life of wild-type p53 in contrast to mutated p53, immunodetection of p53 has been interpreted as an indicator of p53 mutations. However, besides studies showing a good correlation between immune reaction and mutational analysis, others did not observe any correlation[114, 115]. Mutated p53 is found in more than 50% of all tumours and constitutes an important step in tumourigenesis.

5.2.1.3 IS MMP-13 EXPRESSION INDUCED BY MUTANT P53?

It has been previously reported that different factors such as IL-1, TNF-α, TGF-β, KGF, bFGF, aFGF, PDGF and EGF can induce MMP-13 expression in different tumours[107, 116]. It is noteworthy that wild-type p53 was observed to repress MMP-13 promotor. This effect could be reversed by overexpression of some *TP53* mutants (p53Ala^{143}, p53Trp^{248}, p53His^{273} and p53 Gly^{281}). The p53Gly^{281} mutant, a "gain of function" mutant, not only lost its repression function but also stimulated MMP-13 promotor up to 2-3- fold[76]. Thus, adenoviral delivery of wild-type p53 resulted in potent inhibition (71% to 92%) of proMMP-13 production[117]. Based on these observations we hypothesised that specific *TP*53 mutants may lead to induction of MMP-13 expression in MPNST, and therefore screened 36 MPNST for *TP53* mutations.

Screening for *TP53* mutations

Although previous studies reported that MPNST carry *TP53* mutations, the proportion of MPNST carrying *TP53* mutants differs strongly among them (0-100%)[114, 118-122]. *TP53* mutation analysis of MPNST reported until now generally screened a limited number of *TP53* exons in small panels of MPNST (Table 16).

Table 16: *TP*53 mutation analysis previously performed in MPNST

Examined Region	TP53 mut/ MPNST	%	NF1 Patients	References
Exon 4-9	1/1	100	1	Nigro et al. 1989
Exon 4-8	2/7	29	7	Menon et al. 1990
Exon 4-9	2/3	67	3	Legius et al. 1994
Exon 5-9	1/9	11	Unknown	Castresana et al. 1995
Exon 2-11	0/16	0	11	Lothe et al. 2001
Exon 5-8	7/25	28	11	Birindelli et al. 2001
Exon 5-8	1/12	8	2	Mawrin et al. 2002

We found *TP53* mutants in 11 % of MPNST indicating that functional p53 inactivation rarely contributes to their development. Though rare, *TP53* mutations may be of major importance in the development of individual tumours that contain them. This is supported by the fact that *TP53/NF1* haploinsuficient mice develop MPNST like tumours[123, 124]. However, MPNST are uncommon in mice and humans with hereditary defects in *TP53* (Li-Fraumeni Syndrome). Although all tumours with a *TP53* mutation had p53 accumulation, the vast majority of tumours positive for p53 carried wild-type *TP53*. P53 positivity without an underlying mutation suggests an altered turnover of p53. P53 overexpression or impaired degradation leads to protein accumulation. Thus, the presence of unidentified p53-interacting proteins, induced by cellular stress like hypoxia, may contribute to p53 stabilization. On the other hand, at least 25% of the tumour population must carry the mutation to allow detection by direct sequencing[125].

A highly significant association was observed between the expression of MMP-13 and p53 in MPNST. This association was still significant after taking into account the different levels of MMP-13 and p53 expression (p=0.02, Pearson correlation). However, mutant *TP53* was observed in only 11% MPNST and none of the 4 different mutants observed have been functionally described until now. Though all MPNST harbouring *TP53* mutations expressed MMP-13, 20 tumours with wild type *TP53* also expressed MMP-13 indicating that *TP53* mutants are not the major player in MMP-13 induction.

5.2.1.4 CLINICAL RELEVANCE OF MMP-13 EXPRESSION AND P53 STATUS IN MPNST PATIENTS

We included 36 patients in this study to assess the clinical relevance of MMP-13 and p53 mutation states and expression in MPNST. Twenty-four patients were diagnosed with NF1. The mean time of follow-up was 41 months. Tumours were located predominantly in the trunk. Nevertheless, peripheral location of MPNST, allowing a more aggressive surgery, was significantly associated with better prognosis and longer survival. Recurrence was observed in about 45% of patients after a mean time of 18 months. Metastatic spreading occurred in about 39% of patients, located predominantly in the lungs. The 5 year survival rate was 16.7%.

One aim of this study was to assess differences in the clinical course and prognosis between NF1 and non-NF1-associated MPNST. In this regard, NF1 patients develop MPNST at a younger age (32.6 years) than non-NF1 patients. This observation was already made by other groups[16, 66, 126]. Skin of NF1 patients already carries a somatic NF1 allele inactivation. pNF are thought to carry an inactivation of the second allele in a Schwann cell precursor population and will need other genetic aberrations to progress to an MPNST. As sporadic MPNST arise "de novo" over a healthy skin, it is obvious that it will need a longer time to allow genetic alterations to occur. Some studies point out that NF1 patients have a more aggressive clinical course than sporadic MPNST[126]. However, in our study no significant differences were observed in sex prevalence, tumour grading, relapse, metastasis and overall survival between both groups. If both kinds of MPNST share the same pathogenic mechanisms remains unclear. However, microarray analysis failed to find a gene expression profile able to discriminate between NF1-associated and sporadic MPNST. The lack of expression differences might support the hypothesis of similar genetic and epigenetic alterations in both groups of MPNST.

Clinical relevance of MMP-13 expression in MPNST patients

A major aim of this study was to assess the prognostic relevance of MMP-13 expression in MPNST. Tumours expressing MMP-13 were observed to relapse more frequently and earlier than MMP-13 negative tumours. Thus, the risk of relapsing increases with higher levels of MMP-13.

Our results clearly indicate that MMP-13 expression contributes to the recurrent behaviour of MPNST. Absence of MMP-13 expression in healthy adult tissues makes MMP-13 an attractive therapeutic target. However, clinical trials of broad-spectrum MMP inhibitors were disappointing until now[127-131]. Refined strategies to block specific tumour-associated pro-MMPs or to specifically cleave MMP-13 transcripts by using the ribozyme-based therapy are currently under consideration. More specific MMP inhibitors in combination with conventional chemotherapy are thought to yield better response rates.

Clinical relevance of p53 sequence alterations in MPNST patients

Tumours carrying a mutation in p53 showed a more aggressive histology: all tumours were grade 3 (FNCLCC classification). However, an impact of mutant p53 in survival was not observed, probably due to the paucity of tumours carrying a mutant p53 in our panel.

Frequencies of polymorphic variants of *TP53* were compared with data from controls published in previous studies. Polymorphisms in intron 3 and in exon 4 were compared with a German control group (n=549)[77]. The intron 2 polymorphism was compared to a study containing 154 individuals[78] and the frequency of A^{11992} (intron 3) to Caucasian controls from the NCBI database. No differences in allele distribution were observed between MPNST patient and controls indicating that these polymorphisms are not involved in NF1-associated tumourigenesis. However, p53Pro^{72} was more frequently detected in patients with metastasis (p=0.028; χ^2) and metastasis correlated with reduced survival (p=0.0007, log rank). Polymorphisms in codon 72 (exon 4) have been previously described to show functional differences. Interestingly, the p53Arg^{72} allele was reported to be a better suppressor of cellular transformation [132] and a 5 times better inductor of apoptosis than the p53Pro^{72} allele[133]. Thus, the p53Pro^{72} allele might provide an advantage for metastasis development.

In conclusion, MMP-13 expression appears to contribute to the recurrent behaviour of MPNST and though *TP53* mutations seem not to be very frequent in MPNST, the polymorphic variant p53Pro^{72} might play a role in metastatic spreading. According to these data, analysis of MMP-13 expression and the *TP53* polymorphic variant of codon 72 could be used as markers to identify patients with an increased risk of recurrence and/or metastasis, thereby facilitating decisions on the therapeutic strategy to be applied.

5.2.2 SYNDECAN

The syndecan family of transmembrane proteins (Syn-1 to -4) constitutes a major class of cell surface heparin sulphate proteoglycans. Furthermore, syndecans are essential for increasing the local concentration of growth factors by protecting them from proteolytic cleavage, forming ternary complexes with their receptors and participating in internalisation of ligands[134].

The study of syndecans is of special interest in NF1 patients since it was reported that neurofibromin can bind all 4 syndecan members requiring the transmembrane domain and the proximal-membrane region of the highly conserved cytoplasmatic tail[56]. Furthermore, the C-terminal 4 amino acids (-EFYA) shared by all syndecans interact with CASK that coordinates clustering of receptors and connection to the actin-cytoskeleton by binding to the actin-binding protein 4.1[135, 136]. Neurofibromin, syndecan and CASK have overlapping subcellular distributions and form complexes as evidenced by their coimmunoprecipitation[56]. What is the functional significance of the interaction between neurofibromin and syndecans? Syndecans have a PDZ domain, which usually acts as a molecular scaffold. Therefore, the interaction of neurofibromin with syndecans might be important for the subcellular localisation of neurofibromin which is important for Ras regulation at the cell membrane. However, the exact role of this interaction is not clearly understood.

Therefore, we decided to investigate the protein expression of Syn-1, the most studied, and Syn-4, the most ubiquitously expressed, syndecan in NFs and MPNST[137].

5.2.2.1 SYNDECAN-1

Syn-1 is constitutively expressed on the surface of many mature epithelia and plays an important role in embryogenesis, wound healing, cell-cell adhesion, cell motility, invasiveness as well as in cell proliferation[138-142]. By binding to a variety of secreted growth and differentiation factors at the cell surface, Syn-1 is believed to function as coreceptor for many receptor tyrosine-kinases.

Reduced Syn-1 expression was observed in various cancers including hepatocellular carcinomas[143], gastric cancer[144], laryngeal cancer[145], head and neck carcinoma[146], colorectal carcinoma[147], mesothelioma[148], non-small-cell lung carcinoma[149] and endometrial carcinomas[150] and seemed to correlate with a higher tumour differentiation. In contrast, Syn-1 overexpression was observed in breast carcinomas[151], prostate cancer[152] and pancreatic carcinomas[153] and was associated with aggressive phenotypes and poor prognosis.

Until now, no data has been available concerning Syn-1 expression in NF1-associated tumours. In the present study, Syn-1 expression was examined in 29 peripheral nerve sheath tumours of 21 patients. Approximately 86% of the examined MPNST displayed high Syn-1 expression while NFs did not express Syn-1. Therefore, Syn-1 might be associated with malignant transformation. Interestingly, ectopic expression of Syn-1 in Schwann cells enhances cell spreading by promoting the formation of focal adhesions[154] and actin stress fibers[155]. Transfection of Syn-1 into a squamous cell carcinoma cell line significantly enhances the basal growth and the ability of those cells to form tumours and to metastasise in nude mice[156]. Notably, Syn-1-directed T cells or anti-CD138 immunotoxin[157] have been reported to kill multiple myeloma cells and might therefore be a potential therapeutic strategies in MPNST.

The most striking observation in Syn-1 positive MPNST was increased cytoplasmatic expression in perinuclear vesicles. This pattern of concentrated intracellular Syn-1 has been previously reported in several carcinomas [153, 158-161]. *Burbach et al.* demonstrated that the intracellular vesicles were lysosomes containing surprisingly intact Syn-1[162]. Under normal conditions the cell surface Syn-1 is constitutively endocytated and rapidly degraded in lysosomes. Syn-1 has also been shown to internalise in response to ligands, as demonstrated for Syn-1-lipoprotein lipase[163]. As ECM proteins are also degraded in lysosomes of invasive cells[164], Syn-1 could act as a receptor or chaperone for the internalisation and delivery of matrix material through the endosomes to lysosomes for destruction. However, further studies are needed to elucidate the specific cellular function of Syn-1.

5.2.2.2 SYNDECAN-4

In adults Syn-4 is expressed in liver, kidney and lung while the heart and brain show moderate expression[134, 165, 166].

By binding directly to FGF-2, Syn-4 increases the affinity of FGF-2 for its receptor and mediates cell proliferation[167]. Syn-4 has also been proven to be the proteoglycan responsible for focal adhesion formation in response to fibronectin[168, 169]. While Syn-4 overexpression generates an enhanced adhesive phenotype that prevents migration, loss of Syn-4 results in impaired focal adhesion turnover[170]. Optimal levels of Syn-4 seem to be required for efficient migration. Altered Syn-4 expression has been observed in the skin after incisional wounding[171] and in carotid artery tissue after balloon-catheter injury of the vascular SMCs[172].

In our study tumours cells of only one pNF expressed Syn-4. However, the most striking observation was a significant reduction of Syn-4 expression by SMCs around arteries and arterioles in MPNST. Furthermore, benign tumours appeared to be more vascularised and contain blood vessels with increased diameter and intimal hyperplasia. In contrast, MPNST seemed to have a reduced ability to form arterioles as they showed blood vessels with small diameter and thin walls. These observations are in agreement with previous studies showing an impaired angiogenesis, a significant reduction of vessel size and delayed wound repair in Syn-4$^{-/-}$ mice[173].

Syn-4 is proposed to function as an anti-migratory/anti-invasive-signal in cancer cells as Syn-4 is downregulated in colon carcinoma cells[174, 175] and blockage of Syn-4 ligation by tenascin-C increased glioblastoma and breast cancer migration[176]. As Syn-4 plays a crucial role in focal adhesion complex assembly and in cell migration, a reduction of Syn-4 expression by SMCs in MPNST might play a role in NF1-tumourigenesis.

5.2.3 PLATELET DERIVED GROWTH FACTOR RECEPTOR ALPHA

Platelet-derived growth factor receptors (PDGFRs) are implicated in the regulation of proliferation, migration, transformation and apoptosis[177-179]. PDGF receptors, PDGFR-α and -β, are cell surface tyrosine-kinase receptors that exert their cellular effects by dimerisation and subsequent autophosphorylation. The α-receptor binds 4 dimeric isoforms of PDGF (PDGF AA, AB, BB and CC), whereas the β-receptors binds PDGF BB and DD[180-183]. Platelet-derived growth factors (PDGFs) are among the most potent stimuli for mesenchymal cell migration[184] and play an important role in wound healing, inflammation and angiogenesis. Expression studies in brain tumours of PDGF ligands and receptors, including PDGF-A, PDGFR-α and PDGFR-β, have shown that their overexpression occurs in high-grade gliomas[185-188]. Furthermore, overexpression of PDGFR-α seems to be particularly common in tumours of the oligodendroglial lineage with high expression in 100% of tumours studied by IHC[189, 190]. In addition, PDGFR-α was observed to be differentially expressed in bone tumours: osteosarcomas showed a higher expression than osteoblastomas[191]. Similarly, prostate adenocarcinoma and invasive breast cancer have also shown high expression of PDGFR-α[191].

In NF1-associated tumours, PDGFR-α was identified to be differentially expressed between a pNF and an MPNST by SSH. The level of PDGFR-α expression was 15-folds higher in MPNST[74]. Furthermore, previous IHC stainings performed at the Institute of Neuropathology showed that PDGFR-alpha was strongly expressed in 100% of MPNST (n= 16) but was also positive, although less pronounced, in 83 % of benign NFs (n=18) [74].

By WB analysis, 50% MPNST (3/6), an MPNST cell culture and a pNF showed a 185 kDa band corresponding to PDGFR-α. This difference could be due to the distinct sensitivity of both methods. By using IHC, tumours with occasional stained cells within the tumour must be considered positive and can not be detected by WB.

High expression of PDGFR-α has been described in several malignancies, however, the mechanisms involved in PDGFR-α overexpression differ in tumour types and can be due to an activating mutation or amplification of the *PDGFRA* gene[184, 192]. PDGFR-α activation is known to increase the proportion of active Ras. In NF1-associated tumours, PDGFR-α overexpression is likely to cause a permanent activation of Ras downstream signalling.

Our study demonstrates overexpression of PDGFR-α in MPNST and in a pNF and validates previous results. This and other studies strongly suggest a role for PDGFR-α in tumourigenesis. This is of great importance because tumours (MPNST or pNF) expressing PDGFR-α could be sensitive to Imatinib mesylate and/or other drugs able to target PDGFR-α.

5.2.5 PRION PROTEIN

Most of the studies on prion protein (PrP) have focused on prion diseases where an abnormal folded isoform of PrP accumulates in the brain. However, the functional role of the normal PrP isoform is not fully understood. A previous study identified by SSH and confirmed by vNB that PrP mRNA was 21-times more strongly expressed in a pNF than in a MPNST of the same patient[74]. In the present study, WB with 16 primary tumours and 2 MPNST cell cultures were performed. PrP was expressed in both dNFs and pNFs, mostly in the monoglycosylated form. However MPNSTs lack PrP expression. These results are in agreement with vNBs and validate PrP expression in NFs on the protein level.

The function of the evolutionary highly conserved PrP is still enigmatic. PrP seems to play a role in neural differentiation[193], lymphocyte proliferation[194], cell adhesion[195] and protection against oxidative stress, as PrP can bind Cu^{++} ions [196, 197] and has superoxide dismutase activity [198, 199]. Furthermore, transgenic mice overexpressing wild-type PrP exhibit degeneration of central and peripheral nerve system as well as skeletal muscle tissue[200]. Interestingly, recent data point to a potential role of PrP in the regulation of apoptosis. Whereas some studies suggest that it protects cells from proapoptotic agents, others found that PrP sensitises cells to undergo apoptosis. *Paitel et al.* showed that PrP regulates p53-dependent caspase 3-mediated neuronal death by upregulation of the p53 promotor transactivation and by downstream of Mdm2 expression[201] (Figure 27). On the other hand, a PrP restricted sequence shares homology with the anti-apoptotic protein Bcl-2[202, 203] and two different cell lines were reported to be protected from apoptosis induced by Bax and serum deprivation mediated by PrP or Bcl-2 expression[204]. Despite results supporting each of these mechanisms, the physiological function(s) might depend on a combination of several factors. Furthermore, PrP might also be involved in cell cycle regulation.

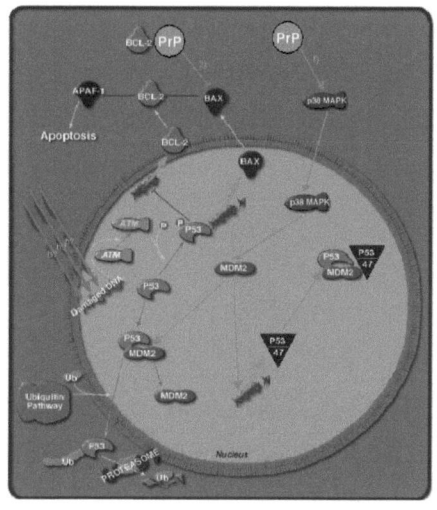

Figure 27: Role of Prion protein in apoptosis: 1) Pro-apoptotic-p53-dependent activity of PrP; 2) anti-apoptotic role of PrP.

Several cell lines were identified to express high levels of PrP when they were arrested in G1 phase[205]. It is noteworthy that p53 is also involved in the checkpoint at the G1/S stage of the cell cycle.

To our knowledge, the present work investigates for the first time PrP expression in peripheral nerve sheath tumours. Further studies need to clarify if loss of PrP contributes to a malignant phenotype or if it is a random event, possibly due to dedifferentiation of transformed cells.

5.2.6 PROTEOLIPID PROTEIN

The myelin proteolipid protein (PLP) is a major component of the CNS, expressed mostly in cells of the oligodendrocytic lineage. However, small amounts of *PLP* gene products are synthesised by Schwann cells in the PNS, with DM-20 being the most abundant isoform. PLP/DM-20 is thought to contribute to the compaction and stability of myelin sheaths[206, 207]. Although PLP/DM-20 is not essential for myelin formation[206, 207], overexpression of the *PLP* gene led to demyelination and death of oligodendrocytes[208, 209].

In a previous study, higher levels of *PLP* mRNA were detected in a pNF compared to an MPNST from the same patient. However, we observed, by performing WB with 16 primary tumours, that the highest amount of PLP protein was found in MPNST, especially in both MPNST cell cultures. In contrast, DM-20 was similarly expressed in both NFs and MPNST. While the *PLP* gene promotor tightly regulates which cells express the *PLP* gene, cellular concentration of *PLP* mRNA is regulated by RNA stabilization/destabilization[210, 211]. Therefore, the high levels of *PLP* mRNA observed in NFs by SSH, microarrays and vNB in the absence of detectable protein might be explained by RNA stabilization. The significance of PLP overexpression in MPNST remains unclear.

5.2.7 MATRILIN-2

The matrilin family is characterised by subunits containing von Willebrandt factor A-like domains, which are connected by a variable number of epidermal growth factor-like modules. Little is known about the function and ligand interactions of matrilins in tissues, and most studies have focused on matrilin-1. However, matrilin-2 (mtr-2) is known to be expressed in a variety of tissues, including both loose and dense connective tissues as well as subepithelial basement membranes in skin and digestive tracts. Mtr-2 has been suggested to represent an adaptor protein connecting proteoglycans to the collagen network and, on the other hand, forming collagen independent structures[212].

Although mtr-2 mRNA levels were previously observed to be overexpressed in NFs, on the protein level we did not observe any difference among the different NF1-associated tumours. This strongly suggests regulation of mtr-2 expression at the postransciptional level.

5.2.8 APOLIPOPROTEIN D

Apolipoprotein D (apoD) is a member of the lipocalin family of genes involved in the transport of small hydrophobic molecules[213]. A variety of substances including cholesterol esters[214-216], heme-related metabolites, progesterone and arachidonic acid have been described as putative ligands for this protein. In the PNS, apoD is synthesised by endoneurial fibroblasts[214, 217]. ApoD expression increased up to 500-fold during peripheral nerve regeneration following a lesion in rats[214, 218]. Curiously, in breast and prostate carcinoma cell lines, androgen-induced apoD expression reduced cellular proliferation by 50% [219]. Thus, ApoD has been proposed to be a marker of cell cycle arrest[220]. In contrast, estrogens suppressed apoD expression and stimulated cellular proliferation[221]. Interestingly, under high estrogens conditions such as pregnancy, up to 82% of NF1-female patients experience growth of new NFs or enlargement of existing NFs[222].

In NF1-associated tumours, apoD was firstly identified by SSH to be upregulated in a pNF compared to a MPSNT of the same patient. Microarray analysis also showed higher levels of apoD in NFs than in MPNST. On the protein level, apoD expression was significantly reduced in MPNST. No differences were observed between dNFs and pNFs. Both MPNST cell cultures lacked apoD expression suggesting a protective effect of apoD in NF1-tumourigenesis.

In human breast cancer cells, apoD was reported to induce cell differentiation and lower the cell growth rate[223, 224]. In brain tumours, apoD was proposed to be a marker for low-proliferative, non-infiltrating and potentially curable primary brain tumours[93]. In contrast, apoD negative immunostaining was a predictor of shorter survival in patients with non-resectable prostate cancers[225]. Therefore, apo D expression in NFs suggest a cell differentiation effect in Schwann cells. It will be interesting to perform further investigations in a larger group of patients to assess if apoD expression has a prognostic relevance in NF1-associated peripheral nerve sheath tumours.

6 CONCLUSIONS

Tumourigenesis is a multistep process, involving inactivation of tumour suppressor genes and activation of oncogenes that results in uncontrolled cell growth. MPNST formation requires more than one genetic alteration. Several molecules have been identified to be involved in MPNST formation such as mutant p53[65, 66], CDKN2A[67] and EGF receptor[69].

To identify further genes involved in NF1-tumourigenesis we performed gene expression analysis with 26 primary tumours. 57 genes were identified to be differentially expressed into NF1-associated tumours and hierarchical clustering analysis clearly separated the samples in 3 groups: dNFs, pNFs and MPNST. We pointed out 10 genes best suited to differentiate between dNFs and pNFs (*MALAT-1, UAP-1, MYO10, SEC3L1, APRIN, CYP1B1, NPIP, HSPCA, PABPC3, FJL14803, MTRNR1, NSGX* and *FOS*). No differences in gene expression were observed between NF1-associated and sporadic MPNST. Expression profiling of tumours is a useful tool to improve diagnosis and identify therapeutically relevant molecules that will allow an optimised and individualised treatment of patients.

Recently, several genes have also been identified to be differentially expressed in NF1-associated tumours by RT-PCR[64, 112]. All these different studies provide a large catalogue of genes potentially involved in tumour formation, thereby contributing an important step in the study of NF1-associated tumourigenesis. However, until now, only a few genes were confirmed to be differentially expressed on the protein level. Therefore, the major aim of this study was to verify in primary tumours the expression levels of some of those genes previously identified to be involved in tumour formation of NF1 patients.

In this regard MMP-13, Syn-1 and PDGFR-α were confirmed by WB and IHC and/ or IF to be overexpressed in MPNST. MMP-13, initially identified by SSH[74] and later by RT-PCR[112], was observed to be expressed in 58% of MPNST but not in NFs. Moreover, the expression of this matrix metalloprotease involved in invasion and metastasis was significantly associated with an increased risk of relapse in MPNST patients. As the MMP-13 promotor was shown to be differentially regulated by wild-type and mutant p53[76], we decided to screen MPNST for *TP53* mutations. P53 mutants were found in only 10.5% of MPNST, all of them expressing MMP-13. However many tumours with wild-type *TP53* also expressed MMP-13. MMP-13 expression and p53 accumulation were significantly associated. The p53 polymorphism in codon 72 was identified by sequencing; interestingly the Pro72 allele was associated with delopment of metastases. Syndecans are believed to play a role in cell adhesion, invasion, cell movement and intercellular signalling. The study of syndecans in NF1-associated tumours is of major interest due to their ability to interact with neurofibromin[56]. Ectopic expression of Syn-1 in Schwann cells enhances cell spreading[154]. Transfection of Syn-1 into squamous-cell carcinoma cell line significantly enhanced the basal growth, tumour formation and cell spreading of those cells in nude mice[156]. Interestingly, Syn-1 was overexpressed in 86% MPNST and absent in NFs pointing to a role of Syn-1 in malignant transformation.

WB analyses detected PDGFR-α and PLP expression in 50% of MPNST. PDGFR-α is important in processes such as cell proliferation, transformation and apoptosis[179, 226-228]. PLP is thought to contribute to the compaction and stability of myelin sheaths[206, 207]. However, PLP overexpression leads to impaired myelinisation and death of oligodendrocytes[208, 209].

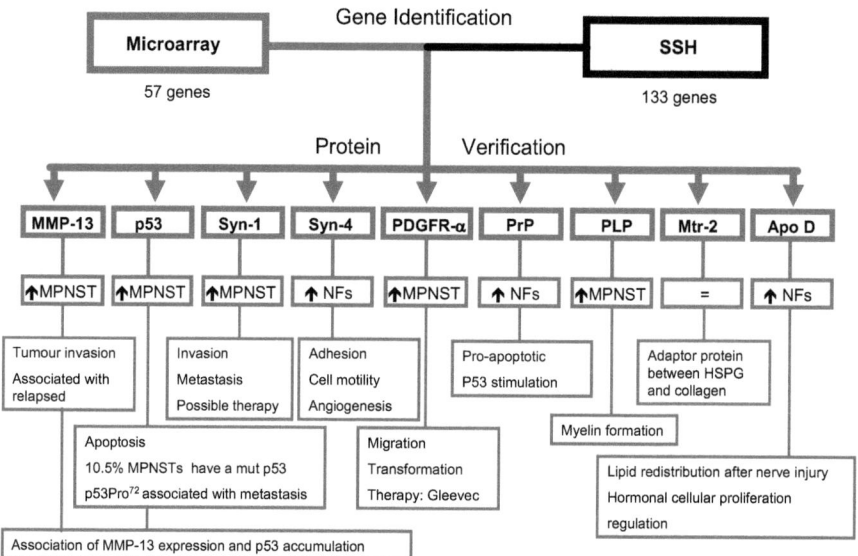

Figure 28: Schematic representation of this work. Firstly, microarray analysis and SSH led to the identification of genes differentially expressed in NF1-associated tumours. I confirmed the differential expression of 9 candidates on the protein level by WB, IHC and/or IF. Furthermore, I assessed the clinical significance of MMP-13 by statistical analysis of MMP-13 expression and *TP53* mutation screening analyses.

The candidates downregulated in MPNST were Syn-4, PrP and apoD. No protein expression differences were observed between NF1-associated tumours for mtr-2. Syn-4 was expressed only by SMCs around arteries and arterioles in NFs and was absent in MPNST which showed small blood vessels with thin walls in comparison to NFs. It is noteworthy that lack of Syn-4 was suggested to be associated with an impaired angiogenesis in Syn-4$^{-/-}$ mice[173]. PrP seems to play a role in neural differentiation, lymphocyte proliferation, cell adhesion and may protect from oxidative stress[194-199]. In addition, several studies point to a function of PrP in cell death and cell cycle[201-204]. All NFs expressed PrP, however most MPNST lacked PrP expression. Impairment of apoptotic signalling due to downregulation of PrP might contribute to malignant transformation of pNFs. ApoD expression was observed to be reduced in MPNST and suggests a protective effect of apoD in NF1-tumourigenesis. Previous studies reported that apoD expression induced cell differentiation and decreased the cell growth rate in human breast cancer cells[223, 224]. In brain tumours, ApoD expression was proposed to be a marker for a group of low-proliferative, non-infiltrating and potentially curable tumours[93].

Therefore, in addition to the model of NF1-peripheral nerve sheath tumourigenesis proposed by Dasgulta and Gutmann, we have verified on the protein level the differential expression of several proteins known to play important roles in tumour formation such as invasion, metastases, angiogenesis, proliferation, cell migration and apoptosis. It is noteworthy that MMP-13 and PDGFR-α are targets of several new therapeutic strategies, already approved or in clinical trials, and constitute a hope for patients with MPNST.

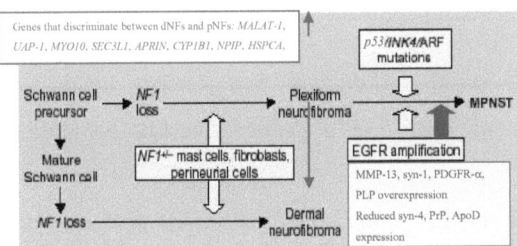

Figure 29: Modified picture from Dasgupta and Gutmann, 2003. New model of NF1-associated peripheral nerve sheath tumourigenesis

This work contributes to partially improving our understanding of the signalling pathways dysregulated in NF1 peripheral nerve sheath tumourigenesis.

7 BIBLIOGRAPHY

1. Easton, D.F., et al., *An analysis of variation in expression of neurofibromatosis (NF) type 1 (NF1): evidence for modifying genes.* Am J Hum Genet, 1993. **53**(2): p. 305-13.
2. Ars, E., et al., *Recurrent mutations in the NF1 gene are common among neurofibromatosis type 1 patients.* J Med Genet, 2003. **40**(6): p. e82.
3. Hyman, S.L., A. Shores, and K.N. North, *The nature and frequency of cognitive deficits in children with neurofibromatosis type 1.* Neurology, 2005. **65**(7): p. 1037-44.
4. Hirsch, N.P., A. Murphy, and J.J. Radcliffe, *Neurofibromatosis: clinical presentations and anaesthetic implications.* Br J Anaesth, 2001. **86**(4): p. 555-64.
5. Zoller, M.E., et al., *Malignant and benign tumors in patients with neurofibromatosis type 1 in a defined Swedish population.* Cancer, 1997. **79**(11): p. 2125-31.
6. Cnossen, M.H., et al., *Endocrinologic disorders and optic pathway gliomas in children with neurofibromatosis type 1.* Pediatrics, 1997. **100**(4): p. 667-70.
7. Hope, D.G. and J.J. Mulvihill, *Malignancy in neurofibromatosis.* Adv Neurol, 1981. **29**: p. 33-56.
8. Carmi, D., et al., *Growth, puberty, and endocrine functions in patients with sporadic or familial neurofibromatosis type 1: a longitudinal study.* Pediatrics, 1999. **103**(6 Pt 1): p. 1257-62.
9. Saxena, K.M., *Endocrine manifestations of neurofibromatosis in children.* Am J Dis Child, 1970. **120**(3): p. 265-71.

10. Szudek, J., P. Birch, and J.M. Friedman, *Growth in North American white children with neurofibromatosis 1 (NF1).* J Med Genet, 2000. **37**(12): p. 933-8.
11. Riccardi, V.M., *Neurofibromatosis: clinical heterogeneity.* Curr Probl Cancer, 1982. **7**(2): p. 1-34.
12. Wolkenstein, P., et al., *More on the frequency of segmental neurofibromatosis.* Arch Dermatol, 1995. **131**(12): p. 1465.
13. Roth, R.R., R. Martines, and W.D. James, *Segmental neurofibromatosis.* Arch Dermatol, 1987. **123**(7): p. 917-20.
14. Reynolds, R.M., et al., *Von Recklinghausen's neurofibromatosis: neurofibromatosis type 1.* Lancet, 2003. **361**(9368): p. 1552-4.
15. Wong, W.W., et al., *Malignant peripheral nerve sheath tumor: analysis of treatment outcome.* Int J Radiat Oncol Biol Phys, 1998. **42**(2): p. 351-60.
16. Evans, D.G., et al., *Malignant peripheral nerve sheath tumours in neurofibromatosis 1.* J Med Genet, 2002. **39**(5): p. 311-4.
17. Tenny, R.T., et al., *The neurosurgical management of optic glioma. Results in 104 patients.* J Neurosurg, 1982. **57**(4): p. 452-8.
18. Parazzini, C., et al., *Spontaneous involution of optic pathway lesions in neurofibromatosis type 1: serial contrast MR evaluation.* AJNR Am J Neuroradiol, 1995. **16**(8): p. 1711-8.
19. Pascual-Castroviejo, I., et al., *[Neurofibromatosis and tumors of the central nervous system (CNS)].* Neurologia, 1986. **1**(1): p. 6-10.
20. Bruni, P., et al., *Solitary intracerebral schwannoma in von Recklinghausen's disease.* Surg Neurol, 1984. **22**(4): p. 360-4.
21. Parizel, P.M., et al., *Cerebral ganglioglioma and neurofibromatosis type I. Case report and review of the literature.* Neuroradiology, 1991. **33**(4): p. 357-9.

22. Cohen, B.H. and A.D. Rothner, *Incidence, types, and management of cancer in patients with neurofibromatosis.* Oncology (Huntingt), 1989. **3**(9): p. 23-30; discussion 34, 37-8.
23. Corkill, A.G. and C.F. Ross, *A case of neurofibromatosis complicated by medulloblastoma, neurogenic sarcoma, and radiation-induced carcinoma of thyroid.* J Neurol Neurosurg Psychiatry, 1969. **32**(1): p. 43-7.
24. Meadows, A.T., et al., *Patterns of second malignant neoplasms in children.* Cancer, 1977. **40**(4 Suppl): p. 1903-11.
25. Poyhonen, M., et al., *Hereditary spinal neurofibromatosis: a rare form of NF1?* J Med Genet, 1997. **34**(3): p. 184-7.
26. Egelhoff, J.C., et al., *Spinal MR findings in neurofibromatosis types 1 and 2.* AJNR Am J Neuroradiol, 1992. **13**(4): p. 1071-7.
27. Mastrangelo, M.J., et al., *Cutaneous melanoma in a patient with neurofibromatosis.* Arch Dermatol, 1979. **115**(7): p. 864-5.
28. Duve, S. and J. Rakoski, *Cutaneous melanoma in a patient with neurofibromatosis: a case report and review of the literature.* Br J Dermatol, 1994. **131**(2): p. 290-4.
29. Specht, C.S. and T.W. Smith, *Uveal malignant melanoma and von Recklinghausen's neurofibromatosis.* Cancer, 1988. **62**(4): p. 812-7.
30. Antle, C.M., et al., *Uveal malignant melanoma and optic nerve glioma in von Recklinghausen's neurofibromatosis.* Br J Ophthalmol, 1990. **74**(8): p. 502-4.
31. Gadner, H. and O.A. Haas, *Experience in pediatric myelodysplastic syndromes.* Hematol Oncol Clin North Am, 1992. **6**(3): p. 655-72.
32. Bader, J.L. and R.W. Miller, *Neurofibromatosis and childhood leukemia.* J Pediatr, 1978. **92**(6): p. 925-9.
33. Shannon, K.M., et al., *Monosomy 7 myeloproliferative disease in children with neurofibromatosis, type 1: epidemiology and molecular analysis.* Blood, 1992. **79**(5): p. 1311-8.

34. Hartley, A.L., et al., *Neurofibromatosis in children with soft tissue sarcoma.* Pediatr Hematol Oncol, 1988. **5**(1): p. 7-16.
35. Walden, P.A., A.G. Johnson, and K.D. Bagshawe, *Wilms's tumour and neurofibromatosis.* Br Med J, 1977. **1**(6064): p. 813.
36. Kindblom, L.G., et al., *Immunohistochemical and molecular analysis of p53, MDM2, proliferating cell nuclear antigen and Ki67 in benign and malignant peripheral nerve sheath tumours.* Virchows Arch, 1995. **427**(1): p. 19-26.
37. Friedman, J.M., *Epidemiology of neurofibromatosis type 1.* Am J Med Genet, 1999. **89**(1): p. 1-6.
38. Stephens, K., et al., *Preferential mutation of the neurofibromatosis type 1 gene in paternally derived chromosomes.* Hum Genet, 1992. **88**(3): p. 279-82.
39. Jadayel, D., et al., *Paternal origin of new mutations in von Recklinghausen neurofibromatosis.* Nature, 1990. **343**(6258): p. 558-9.
40. Riccardi, V.M., et al., *The pathophysiology of neurofibromatosis: IX. Paternal age as a factor in the origin of new mutations.* Am J Med Genet, 1984. **18**(1): p. 169-76.
41. Lazaro, C., et al., *Sex differences in mutational rate and mutational mechanism in the NF1 gene in neurofibromatosis type 1 patients.* Hum Genet, 1996. **98**(6): p. 696-9.
42. Ainsworth, P.J., P.K. Chakraborty, and R. Weksberg, *Example of somatic mosaicism in a series of de novo neurofibromatosis type 1 cases due to a maternally derived deletion.* Hum Mutat, 1997. **9**(5): p. 452-7.
43. Upadhyaya, M., et al., *Gross deletions of the neurofibromatosis type 1 (NF1) gene are predominantly of maternal origin and commonly associated with a learning disability, dysmorphic features and developmental delay.* Hum Genet, 1998. **102**(5): p. 591-7.

44. Feldkamp, M.M., L. Angelov, and A. Guha, *Neurofibromatosis type 1 peripheral nerve tumors: aberrant activation of the Ras pathway.* Surg Neurol, 1999. **51**(2): p. 211-8.
45. Lakkis, M.M., et al., *Neurofibromin deficiency in mice causes exencephaly and is a modifier for Splotch neural tube defects.* Dev Biol, 1999. **212**(1): p. 80-92.
46. Guo, H.F., et al., *Requirement of Drosophila NF1 for activation of adenylyl cyclase by PACAP38-like neuropeptides.* Science, 1997. **276**(5313): p. 795-8.
47. The, I., et al., *Rescue of a Drosophila NF1 mutant phenotype by protein kinase A.* Science, 1997. **276**(5313): p. 791-4.
48. Gregory, P.E., et al., *Neurofibromatosis type 1 gene product (neurofibromin) associates with microtubules.* Somat Cell Mol Genet, 1993. **19**(3): p. 265-74.
49. Bollag, G., F. McCormick, and R. Clark, *Characterization of full-length neurofibromin: tubulin inhibits Ras GAP activity.* Embo J, 1993. **12**(5): p. 1923-7.
50. Hakimi, M.A., D.W. Speicher, and R. Shiekhattar, *The motor protein kinesin-1 links neurofibromin and merlin in a common cellular pathway of neurofibromatosis.* J Biol Chem, 2002. **277**(40): p. 36909-12.
51. Hirokawa, N., Y. Noda, and Y. Okada, *Kinesin and dynein superfamily proteins in organelle transport and cell division.* Curr Opin Cell Biol, 1998. **10**(1): p. 60-73.
52. Brendza, K.M., et al., *A kinesin mutation that uncouples motor domains and desensitizes the gamma-phosphate sensor.* J Biol Chem, 2000. **275**(29): p. 22187-95.
53. Zhu, Y., et al., *Ablation of NF1 function in neurons induces abnormal development of cerebral cortex and reactive gliosis in the brain.* Genes Dev, 2001. **15**(7): p. 859-76.
54. Zhu, Y. and L.F. Parada, *Neurofibromin, a tumor suppressor in the nervous system.* Exp Cell Res, 2001. **264**(1): p. 19-28.

55. Costa, R.M., et al., *Mechanism for the learning deficits in a mouse model of neurofibromatosis type 1.* Nature, 2002. **415**(6871): p. 526-30.
56. Hsueh, Y.P., et al., *Bipartite interaction between neurofibromatosis type I protein (neurofibromin) and syndecan transmembrane heparan sulfate proteoglycans.* J Neurosci, 2001. **21**(11): p. 3764-70.
57. Knudson, A.G., Jr., *Genetic predisposition to cancer.* Cancer Detect Prev, 1984. **7**(1): p. 1-8.
58. Rutkowski, J.L., et al., *Genetic and cellular defects contributing to benign tumor formation in neurofibromatosis type 1.* Hum Mol Genet, 2000. **9**(7): p. 1059-66.
59. Perry, A., et al., *NF1 deletions in S-100 protein-positive and negative cells of sporadic and neurofibromatosis 1 (NF1)-associated plexiform neurofibromas and malignant peripheral nerve sheath tumors.* Am J Pathol, 2001. **159**(1): p. 57-61.
60. Arun, D. and D.H. Gutmann, *Recent advances in neurofibromatosis type 1.* Curr Opin Neurol, 2004. **17**(2): p. 101-5.
61. Ling, B.C., et al., *Role for the epidermal growth factor receptor in neurofibromatosis-related peripheral nerve tumorigenesis.* Cancer Cell, 2005. **7**(1): p. 65-75.
62. Cappione, A.J., B.L. French, and G.R. Skuse, *A potential role for NF1 mRNA editing in the pathogenesis of NF1 tumors.* Am J Hum Genet, 1997. **60**(2): p. 305-12.
63. De Raedt, T., et al., *Elevated risk for MPNST in NF1 microdeletion patients.* Am J Hum Genet, 2003. **72**(5): p. 1288-92.
64. Levy, P., et al., *Molecular profiles of neurofibromatosis type 1-associated plexiform neurofibromas: identification of a gene expression signature of poor prognosis.* Clin Cancer Res, 2004. **10**(11): p. 3763-71.

65. Halling, K.C., et al., *p53 expression in neurofibroma and malignant peripheral nerve sheath tumor. An immunohistochemical study of sporadic and NF1-associated tumors.* Am J Clin Pathol, 1996. **106**(3): p. 282-8.
66. Ducatman, B.S., et al., *Malignant peripheral nerve sheath tumors. A clinicopathologic study of 120 cases.* Cancer, 1986. **57**(10): p. 2006-21.
67. Kourea, H.P., et al., *Deletions of the INK4A gene occur in malignant peripheral nerve sheath tumors but not in neurofibromas.* Am J Pathol, 1999. **155**(6): p. 1855-60.
68. Kourea, H.P., et al., *Expression of p27(kip) and other cell cycle regulators in malignant peripheral nerve sheath tumors and neurofibromas: the emerging role of p27(kip) in malignant transformation of neurofibromas.* Am J Pathol, 1999. **155**(6): p. 1885-91.
69. DeClue, J.E., et al., *Epidermal growth factor receptor expression in neurofibromatosis type 1-related tumors and NF1 animal models.* J Clin Invest, 2000. **105**(9): p. 1233-41.
70. Perry, A., et al., *Differential NF1, p16, and EGFR patterns by interphase cytogenetics (FISH) in malignant peripheral nerve sheath tumor (MPNST) and morphologically similar spindle cell neoplasms.* J Neuropathol Exp Neurol, 2002. **61**(8): p. 702-9.
71. Miller, S.J., et al., *Brain lipid binding protein in axon-Schwann cell interactions and peripheral nerve tumorigenesis.* Mol Cell Biol, 2003. **23**(6): p. 2213-24.
72. Su, W., et al., *Malignant peripheral nerve sheath tumor cell invasion is facilitated by Src and aberrant CD44 expression.* Glia, 2003. **42**(4): p. 350-8.
73. Gutmann, D.H., *New insights into the neurofibromatoses.* Curr Opin Neurol, 1994. **7**(2): p. 166-71.

74. Holtkamp, N., et al., *Differentially expressed genes in neurofibromatosis 1-associated neurofibromas and malignant peripheral nerve sheath tumors.* Acta Neuropathol (Berl), 2004. **107**(2): p. 159-68.
75. Holtkamp, N., et al., *Subclassification of nerve sheath tumors by gene expression profiling.* Brain Pathol, 2004. **14**(3): p. 258-64.
76. Sun, Y., et al., *Wild type and mutant p53 differentially regulate the gene expression of human collagenase-3 (hMMP-13).* J Biol Chem, 2000. **275**(15): p. 11327-32.
77. Wang-Gohrke, S., et al., *Intron 3 16 bp duplication polymorphism of p53 is associated with an increased risk for breast cancer by the age of 50 years.* Pharmacogenetics, 2002. **12**(3): p. 269-72.
78. Verselis, S.J. and F.P. Li, *Common polymorphism in p53 intron 2, IVS2+38G>C.* Hum Mutat, 2000. **16**(2): p. 181.
79. Grutzmann, R., et al., *ADAM9 expression in pancreatic cancer is associated with tumour type and is a prognostic factor in ductal adenocarcinoma.* Br J Cancer, 2004. **90**(5): p. 1053-8.
80. Cerutti, J.M., et al., *A preoperative diagnostic test that distinguishes benign from malignant thyroid carcinoma based on gene expression.* J Clin Invest, 2004. **113**(8): p. 1234-42.
81. Murray, G.I., et al., *Tumor-specific expression of cytochrome P450 CYP1B1.* Cancer Res, 1997. **57**(14): p. 3026-31.
82. Murray, G.I., et al., *Regulation, function, and tissue-specific expression of cytochrome P450 CYP1B1.* Annu Rev Pharmacol Toxicol, 2001. **41**: p. 297-316.
83. Rochat, B., et al., *Human CYP1B1 and anticancer agent metabolism: mechanism for tumor-specific drug inactivation?* J Pharmacol Exp Ther, 2001. **296**(2): p. 537-41.

84. Ji, P., et al., *MALAT-1, a novel noncoding RNA, and thymosin beta4 predict metastasis and survival in early-stage non-small cell lung cancer.* Oncogene, 2003. **22**(39): p. 8031-41.
85. Weber, K.L., et al., *A microtubule-binding myosin required for nuclear anchoring and spindle assembly.* Nature, 2004. **431**(7006): p. 325-9.
86. Zhang, H., et al., *Myosin-X provides a motor-based link between integrins and the cytoskeleton.* Nat Cell Biol, 2004. **6**(6): p. 523-31.
87. Maiguel, D.A., et al., *Nucleophosmin sets a threshold for p53 response to UV radiation.* Mol Cell Biol, 2004. **24**(9): p. 3703-11.
88. Cunningham, D., et al., *Cetuximab monotherapy and cetuximab plus irinotecan in irinotecan-refractory metastatic colorectal cancer.* N Engl J Med, 2004. **351**(4): p. 337-45.
89. Noble, M.E., J.A. Endicott, and L.N. Johnson, *Protein kinase inhibitors: insights into drug design from structure.* Science, 2004. **303**(5665): p. 1800-5.
90. Ranson, M., et al., *ZD1839, a selective oral epidermal growth factor receptor-tyrosine kinase inhibitor, is well tolerated and active in patients with solid, malignant tumors: results of a phase I trial.* J Clin Oncol, 2002. **20**(9): p. 2240-50.
91. Yarden, R.I., M.A. Wilson, and S.A. Chrysogelos, *Estrogen suppression of EGFR expression in breast cancer cells: a possible mechanism to modulate growth.* J Cell Biochem Suppl, 2001. **Suppl 36**: p. 232-46.
92. Peek, R., et al., *The angiopoietin-like factor cornea-derived transcript 6 is a putative morphogen for human cornea.* J Biol Chem, 2002. **277**(1): p. 686-93.
93. Hunter, S., et al., *Differential expression between pilocytic and anaplastic astrocytomas: identification of apolipoprotein D as a marker for low-grade, non-infiltrating primary CNS neoplasms.* J Neuropathol Exp Neurol, 2002. **61**(3): p. 275-81.

94. Aspinall, J.O., et al., *Differential expression of apolipoprotein-D and prostate specific antigen in benign and malignant prostate tissues*. J Urol, 1995. **154**(2 Pt 1): p. 622-8.
95. Quarles, R.H., *Myelin sheaths: glycoproteins involved in their formation, maintenance and degeneration*. Cell Mol Life Sci, 2002. **59**(11): p. 1851-71.
96. Greer, J.M., et al., *Thiopalmitoylation of myelin proteolipid protein epitopes enhances immunogenicity and encephalitogenicity*. J Immunol, 2001. **166**(11): p. 6907-13.
97. Xu, N., C.Y. Chen, and A.B. Shyu, *Modulation of the fate of cytoplasmic mRNA by AU-rich elements: key sequence features controlling mRNA deadenylation and decay*. Mol Cell Biol, 1997. **17**(8): p. 4611-21.
98. Mitchell, P.G., et al., *Cloning, expression, and type II collagenolytic activity of matrix metalloproteinase-13 from human osteoarthritic cartilage*. J Clin Invest, 1996. **97**(3): p. 761-8.
99. Knauper, V., et al., *Biochemical characterization of human collagenase-3*. J Biol Chem, 1996. **271**(3): p. 1544-50.
100. Ashworth, J.L., et al., *Fibrillin degradation by matrix metalloproteinases: implications for connective tissue remodelling*. Biochem J, 1999. **340 (Pt 1)**: p. 171-81.
101. Pagenstecher, A., et al., *Differential expression of matrix metalloproteinase and tissue inhibitor of matrix metalloproteinase genes in the mouse central nervous system in normal and inflammatory states*. Am J Pathol, 1998. **152**(3): p. 729-41.
102. Vaalamo, M., et al., *Distinct expression profiles of stromelysin-2 (MMP-10), collagenase-3 (MMP-13), macrophage metalloelastase (MMP-12), and tissue inhibitor of metalloproteinases-3 (TIMP-3) in intestinal ulcerations*. Am J Pathol, 1998. **152**(4): p. 1005-14.

103. Uitto, V.J., et al., *Collagenase-3 (matrix metalloproteinase-13) expression is induced in oral mucosal epithelium during chronic inflammation.* Am J Pathol, 1998. **152**(6): p. 1489-99.
104. Sukhova, G.K., et al., *Evidence for increased collagenolysis by interstitial collagenases-1 and -3 in vulnerable human atheromatous plaques.* Circulation, 1999. **99**(19): p. 2503-9.
105. Zijlstra, A., et al., *Collagenolysis-dependent angiogenesis mediated by matrix metalloproteinase-13 (collagenase-3).* J Biol Chem, 2004. **279**(26): p. 27633-45.
106. Freije, J.M., et al., *Molecular cloning and expression of collagenase-3, a novel human matrix metalloproteinase produced by breast carcinomas.* J Biol Chem, 1994. **269**(24): p. 16766-73.
107. Uria, J.A., et al., *Regulation of collagenase-3 expression in human breast carcinomas is mediated by stromal-epithelial cell interactions.* Cancer Res, 1997. **57**(21): p. 4882-8.
108. Johansson, N., et al., *Expression of collagenase-3 (matrix metalloproteinase-13) in squamous cell carcinomas of the head and neck.* Am J Pathol, 1997. **151**(2): p. 499-508.
109. Cazorla, M., et al., *Collagenase-3 expression is associated with advanced local invasion in human squamous cell carcinomas of the larynx.* J Pathol, 1998. **186**(2): p. 144-50.
110. Airola, K., et al., *Human collagenase-3 is expressed in malignant squamous epithelium of the skin.* J Invest Dermatol, 1997. **109**(2): p. 225-31.
111. Johansson, N., et al., *Collagenase-3 (MMP-13) is expressed by tumor cells in invasive vulvar squamous cell carcinomas.* Am J Pathol, 1999. **154**(2): p. 469-80.

112. Levy, P., et al., *Molecular profiling of malignant peripheral nerve sheath tumors associated with neurofibromatosis type 1, based on large-scale real-time RT-PCR.* Mol Cancer, 2004. **3**(1): p. 20.
113. Johansson, N., et al., *Expression of collagenase-3 (MMP-13) and collagenase-1 (MMP-1) by transformed keratinocytes is dependent on the activity of p38 mitogen-activated protein kinase.* J Cell Sci, 2000. **113 Pt 2**: p. 227-35.
114. Mawrin, C., et al., *Immunohistochemical and molecular analysis of p53, RB, and PTEN in malignant peripheral nerve sheath tumors.* Virchows Arch, 2002. **440**(6): p. 610-5.
115. Battifora, H., *p53 immunohistochemistry: a word of caution.* Hum Pathol, 1994. **25**(5): p. 435-7.
116. Balbin, M., et al., *Expression and regulation of collagenase-3 (MMP-13) in human malignant tumors.* Apmis, 1999. **107**(1): p. 45-53.
117. Ala-aho, R., et al., *Adenoviral delivery of p53 gene suppresses expression of collagenase-3 (MMP-13) in squamous carcinoma cells.* Oncogene, 2002. **21**(8): p. 1187-95.
118. Menon, A.G., et al., *Chromosome 17p deletions and p53 gene mutations associated with the formation of malignant neurofibrosarcomas in von Recklinghausen neurofibromatosis.* Proc Natl Acad Sci U S A, 1990. **87**(14): p. 5435-9.
119. Legius, E., et al., *TP53 mutations are frequent in malignant NF1 tumors.* Genes Chromosomes Cancer, 1994. **10**(4): p. 250-5.
120. Gomez, L., et al., *Absence of mutation at the GAP-related domain of the neurofibromatosis type 1 gene in sporadic neurofibrosarcomas and other bone and soft tissue sarcomas.* Cancer Genet Cytogenet, 1995. **81**(2): p. 173-4.
121. Lothe, R.A., et al., *Biallelic inactivation of TP53 rarely contributes to the development of malignant peripheral nerve sheath tumors.* Genes Chromosomes Cancer, 2001. **30**(2): p. 202-6.

122. Nigro, J.M., et al., *Mutations in the p53 gene occur in diverse human tumour types.* Nature, 1989. **342**(6250): p. 705-8.
123. Cichowski, K., et al., *Mouse models of tumor development in neurofibromatosis type 1.* Science, 1999. **286**(5447): p. 2172-6.
124. Vogel, K.S., et al., *Mouse tumor model for neurofibromatosis type 1.* Science, 1999. **286**(5447): p. 2176-9.
125. Burchill, S.A., D.E. Neal, and J. Lunec, *Frequency of H-ras mutations in human bladder cancer detected by direct sequencing.* Br J Urol, 1994. **73**(5): p. 516-21.
126. Hagel, C., et al., *Histopathology and clinical outcome of NF1-associated vs. sporadic malignant peripheral nerve sheath tumors.* J Neurooncol, 2007. **82**(2): p. 187-92.
127. Brown, P.D., *Ongoing trials with matrix metalloproteinase inhibitors.* Expert Opin Investig Drugs, 2000. **9**(9): p. 2167-77.
128. *Marimastat: BB 2516, TA 2516.* Drugs R D, 2003. **4**(3): p. 198-203.
129. Bonomi, P., *Matrix metalloproteinases and matrix metalloproteinase inhibitors in lung cancer.* Semin Oncol, 2002. **29**(1 Suppl 4): p. 78-86.
130. Sparano, J.A., et al., *Randomized phase III trial of marimastat versus placebo in patients with metastatic breast cancer who have responding or stable disease after first-line chemotherapy: Eastern Cooperative Oncology Group trial E2196.* J Clin Oncol, 2004. **22**(23): p. 4631-8.
131. Bissett, D., et al., *Phase III study of matrix metalloproteinase inhibitor prinomastat in non-small-cell lung cancer.* J Clin Oncol, 2005. **23**(4): p. 842-9.
132. Thomas, M., et al., *Two polymorphic variants of wild-type p53 differ biochemically and biologically.* Mol Cell Biol, 1999. **19**(2): p. 1092-100.
133. Dumont, P., et al., *The codon 72 polymorphic variants of p53 have markedly different apoptotic potential.* Nat Genet, 2003. **33**(3): p. 357-65.

134. Bernfield, M., et al., *Functions of cell surface heparan sulfate proteoglycans.* Annu Rev Biochem, 1999. **68**: p. 729-77.

135. Hsueh, Y.P., et al., *Direct interaction of CASK/LIN-2 and syndecan heparan sulfate proteoglycan and their overlapping distribution in neuronal synapses.* J Cell Biol, 1998. **142**(1): p. 139-51.

136. Bass, M.D. and M.J. Humphries, *Cytoplasmic interactions of syndecan-4 orchestrate adhesion receptor and growth factor receptor signalling.* Biochem J, 2002. **368**(Pt 1): p. 1-15.

137. Gulyas, M. and A. Hjerpe, *Proteoglycans and WT1 as markers for distinguishing adenocarcinoma, epithelioid mesothelioma, and benign mesothelium.* J Pathol, 2003. **199**(4): p. 479-87.

138. Bernfield, M. and R.D. Sanderson, *Syndecan, a developmentally regulated cell surface proteoglycan that binds extracellular matrix and growth factors.* Philos Trans R Soc Lond B Biol Sci, 1990. **327**(1239): p. 171-86.

139. Filla, M.S., P. Dam, and A.C. Rapraeger, *The cell surface proteoglycan syndecan-1 mediates fibroblast growth factor-2 binding and activity.* J Cell Physiol, 1998. **174**(3): p. 310-21.

140. Inki, P. and M. Jalkanen, *The role of syndecan-1 in malignancies.* Ann Med, 1996. **28**(1): p. 63-7.

141. Salmivirta, M. and M. Jalkanen, *Syndecan family of cell surface proteoglycans: developmentally regulated receptors for extracellular effector molecules.* Experientia, 1995. **51**(9-10): p. 863-72.

142. Stanley, M.J., et al., *Heparan sulfate-mediated cell aggregation. Syndecans-1 and -4 mediate intercellular adhesion following their transfection into human B lymphoid cells.* J Biol Chem, 1995. **270**(10): p. 5077-83.

143. Matsumoto, A., et al., *Reduced expression of syndecan-1 in human hepatocellular carcinoma with high metastatic potential.* Int J Cancer, 1997. **74**(5): p. 482-91.

144. Watari, J., et al., *Reduction of syndecan-1 expression in differentiated type early gastric cancer and background mucosa with gastric cellular phenotype.* J Gastroenterol, 2004. **39**(2): p. 104-12.

145. Pulkkinen, J.O., et al., *Syndecan-1: a new prognostic marker in laryngeal cancer.* Acta Otolaryngol, 1997. **117**(2): p. 312-5.

146. Inki, P., et al., *Association between syndecan-1 expression and clinical outcome in squamous cell carcinoma of the head and neck.* Br J Cancer, 1994. **70**(2): p. 319-23.

147. Day, R.M., et al., *Changes in the expression of syndecan-1 in the colorectal adenoma-carcinoma sequence.* Virchows Arch, 1999. **434**(2): p. 121-5.

148. Kumar-Singh, S., et al., *Syndecan-1 expression in malignant mesothelioma: correlation with cell differentiation, WT1 expression, and clinical outcome.* J Pathol, 1998. **186**(3): p. 300-5.

149. Nackaerts, K., et al., *Heparan sulfate proteoglycan expression in human lung-cancer cells.* Int J Cancer, 1997. **74**(3): p. 335-45.

150. Miturski, R., et al., *Immunohistochemical expression of syndecan-1 in human endometrial cancer cells.* Int J Mol Med, 1998. **2**(4): p. 397-401.

151. Barbareschi, M., et al., *High syndecan-1 expression in breast carcinoma is related to an aggressive phenotype and to poorer prognosis.* Cancer, 2003. **98**(3): p. 474-83.

152. Zellweger, T., et al., *Tissue microarray analysis reveals prognostic significance of syndecan-1 expression in prostate cancer.* Prostate, 2003. **55**(1): p. 20-9.

153. Conejo, J.R., et al., *Syndecan-1 expression is up-regulated in pancreatic but not in other gastrointestinal cancers.* Int J Cancer, 2000. **88**(1): p. 12-20.

154. Hansen, C.A., et al., *Localization of a heterotrimeric G protein gamma subunit to focal adhesions and associated stress fibers.* J Cell Biol, 1994. **126**(3): p. 811-9.

155. Febbraio, M.A., et al., *Muscle metabolism during exercise and heat stress in trained men: effect of acclimation.* J Appl Physiol, 1994. **76**(2): p. 589-97.
156. Hirabayashi, K., et al., *Altered proliferative and metastatic potential associated with increased expression of syndecan-1.* Tumour Biol, 1998. **19**(6): p. 454-63.
157. Post, J., et al., *Efficacy of an anti-CD138 immunotoxin and doxorubicin on drug-resistant and drug-sensitive myeloma cells.* Int J Cancer, 1999. **83**(4): p. 571-6.
158. Roskams, T., et al., *Heparan sulphate proteoglycan expression in human primary liver tumours.* J Pathol, 1998. **185**(3): p. 290-7.
159. Stanley, M.J., et al., *Syndecan-1 expression is induced in the stroma of infiltrating breast carcinoma.* Am J Clin Pathol, 1999. **112**(3): p. 377-83.
160. Bayer-Garner, I.B. and B.R. Smoller, *The expression of syndecan-1 is preferentially reduced compared with that of E-cadherin in acantholytic squamous cell carcinoma.* J Cutan Pathol, 2001. **28**(2): p. 83-9.
161. Orosz, Z. and L. Kopper, *Syndecan-1 expression in different soft tissue tumours.* Anticancer Res, 2001. **21**(1B): p. 733-7.
162. Burbach, B.J., et al., *Syndecan-1 accumulates in lysosomes of poorly differentiated breast carcinoma cells.* Matrix Biol, 2003. **22**(2): p. 163-77.
163. Williams, K.J. and I.V. Fuki, *Cell-surface heparan sulfate proteoglycans: dynamic molecules mediating ligand catabolism.* Curr Opin Lipidol, 1997. **8**(5): p. 253-62.
164. Sameni, M., K. Moin, and B.F. Sloane, *Imaging proteolysis by living human breast cancer cells.* Neoplasia, 2000. **2**(6): p. 496-504.
165. Carey, D.J., *Syndecans: multifunctional cell-surface co-receptors.* Biochem J, 1997. **327 (Pt 1)**: p. 1-16.
166. Kim, C.W., et al., *Members of the syndecan family of heparan sulfate proteoglycans are expressed in distinct cell-, tissue-, and development-specific patterns.* Mol Biol Cell, 1994. **5**(7): p. 797-805.

167. Richardson, T.P., V. Trinkaus-Randall, and M.A. Nugent, *Regulation of basic fibroblast growth factor binding and activity by cell density and heparan sulfate.* J Biol Chem, 1999. **274**(19): p. 13534-40.

168. Longley, R.L., et al., *Control of morphology, cytoskeleton and migration by syndecan-4.* J Cell Sci, 1999. **112 (Pt 20)**: p. 3421-31.

169. Baciu, P.C. and P.F. Goetinck, *Protein kinase C regulates the recruitment of syndecan-4 into focal contacts.* Mol Biol Cell, 1995. **6**(11): p. 1503-13.

170. Wilcox-Adelman, S.A., et al., *Syndecan-4: dispensable or indispensable?* Glycoconj J, 2002. **19**(4-5): p. 305-13.

171. Gallo, R., et al., *Syndecans-1 and -4 are induced during wound repair of neonatal but not fetal skin.* J Invest Dermatol, 1996. **107**(5): p. 676-83.

172. Cizmeci-Smith, G., et al., *Syndecan-4 is a primary-response gene induced by basic fibroblast growth factor and arterial injury in vascular smooth muscle cells.* Arterioscler Thromb Vasc Biol, 1997. **17**(1): p. 172-80.

173. Echtermeyer, F., et al., *Delayed wound repair and impaired angiogenesis in mice lacking syndecan-4.* J Clin Invest, 2001. **107**(2): p. R9-R14.

174. Jayson, G.C., et al., *Coordinated modulation of the fibroblast growth factor dual receptor mechanism during transformation from human colon adenoma to carcinoma.* Int J Cancer, 1999. **82**(2): p. 298-304.

175. Park, H., et al., *Syndecan-2 mediates adhesion and proliferation of colon carcinoma cells.* J Biol Chem, 2002. **277**(33): p. 29730-6.

176. Huang, W., et al., *Interference of tenascin-C with syndecan-4 binding to fibronectin blocks cell adhesion and stimulates tumor cell proliferation.* Cancer Res, 2001. **61**(23): p. 8586-94.

177. Eriksson, A., et al., *PDGF alpha- and beta-receptors activate unique and common signal transduction pathways.* Embo J, 1992. **11**(2): p. 543-50.

178. Keating, M.T., C.C. Harryman, and L.T. Williams, *Platelet-derived growth factor receptor inducibility is acquired immediately after translation and does not require glycosylation.* J Biol Chem, 1989. **264**(16): p. 9129-32.

179. Shinbrot, E., K.G. Peters, and L.T. Williams, *Expression of the platelet-derived growth factor beta receptor during organogenesis and tissue differentiation in the mouse embryo.* Dev Dyn, 1994. **199**(3): p. 169-75.

180. Matsui, T., et al., *Independent expression of human alpha or beta platelet-derived growth factor receptor cDNAs in a naive hematopoietic cell leads to functional coupling with mitogenic and chemotactic signaling pathways.* Proc Natl Acad Sci U S A, 1989. **86**(21): p. 8314-8.

181. Nister, M., et al., *Expression of messenger RNAs for platelet-derived growth factor and transforming growth factor-alpha and their receptors in human malignant glioma cell lines.* Cancer Res, 1988. **48**(14): p. 3910-8.

182. Claesson-Welsh, L., *Mechanism of action of platelet-derived growth factor.* Int J Biochem Cell Biol, 1996. **28**(4): p. 373-85.

183. Gronwald, R.G., et al., *Cloning and expression of a cDNA coding for the human platelet-derived growth factor receptor: evidence for more than one receptor class.* Proc Natl Acad Sci U S A, 1988. **85**(10): p. 3435-9.

184. Clarke, I.D. and P.B. Dirks, *A human brain tumor-derived PDGFR-alpha deletion mutant is transforming.* Oncogene, 2003. **22**(5): p. 722-33.

185. Redwine, J.M. and R.C. Armstrong, *In vivo proliferation of oligodendrocyte progenitors expressing PDGFalphaR during early remyelination.* J Neurobiol, 1998. **37**(3): p. 413-28.

186. Nister, M., et al., *Differential expression of platelet-derived growth factor receptors in human malignant glioma cell lines.* J Biol Chem, 1991. **266**(25): p. 16755-63.

187. Fleming, T.P., et al., *Amplification and/or overexpression of platelet-derived growth factor receptors and epidermal growth factor receptor in human glial tumors.* Cancer Res, 1992. **52**(16): p. 4550-3.
188. Kumabe, T., et al., *Overexpression and amplification of alpha-PDGF receptor gene lacking exons coding for a portion of the extracellular region in a malignant glioma.* Tohoku J Exp Med, 1992. **168**(2): p. 265-9.
189. Di Rocco, F., et al., *Platelet-derived growth factor and its receptor expression in human oligodendrogliomas.* Neurosurgery, 1998. **42**(2): p. 341-6.
190. Shoshan, Y., et al., *Expression of oligodendrocyte progenitor cell antigens by gliomas: implications for the histogenesis of brain tumors.* Proc Natl Acad Sci U S A, 1999. **96**(18): p. 10361-6.
191. Sulzbacher, I., et al., *Platelet-derived growth factor-AA and -alpha receptor expression suggests an autocrine and/or paracrine loop in osteosarcoma.* Mod Pathol, 2000. **13**(6): p. 632-7.
192. Galanis, E., et al., *Gene amplification as a prognostic factor in primary and secondary high-grade malignant gliomas.* Int J Oncol, 1998. **13**(4): p. 717-24.
193. Mobley, W.C., et al., *Nerve growth factor increases mRNA levels for the prion protein and the beta-amyloid protein precursor in developing hamster brain.* Proc Natl Acad Sci U S A, 1988. **85**(24): p. 9811-5.
194. Cashman, N.R., et al., *Cellular isoform of the scrapie agent protein participates in lymphocyte activation.* Cell, 1990. **61**(1): p. 185-92.
195. Stamatoglou, S.C., et al., *Temporal changes in the expression and distribution of adhesion molecules during liver development and regeneration.* J Cell Biol, 1992. **116**(6): p. 1507-15.
196. Hornshaw, M.P., J.R. McDermott, and J.M. Candy, *Copper binding to the N-terminal tandem repeat regions of mammalian and avian prion protein.* Biochem Biophys Res Commun, 1995. **207**(2): p. 621-9.

197. Stockel, J., et al., *Prion protein selectively binds copper(II) ions*. Biochemistry, 1998. **37**(20): p. 7185-93.
198. Brown, D.R., et al., *The cellular prion protein binds copper in vivo*. Nature, 1997. **390**(6661): p. 684-7.
199. Brown, D.R., et al., *Prion protein-deficient cells show altered response to oxidative stress due to decreased SOD-1 activity*. Exp Neurol, 1997. **146**(1): p. 104-12.
200. Brown, D.R., et al., *Prion protein expression in muscle cells and toxicity of a prion protein fragment*. Eur J Cell Biol, 1998. **75**(1): p. 29-37.
201. Paitel, E., R. Fahraeus, and F. Checler, *Cellular prion protein sensitizes neurons to apoptotic stimuli through Mdm2-regulated and p53-dependent caspase 3-like activation*. J Biol Chem, 2003. **278**(12): p. 10061-6.
202. Yin, X.M., et al., *Bcl-2 gene family and the regulation of programmed cell death*. Cold Spring Harb Symp Quant Biol, 1994. **59**: p. 387-93.
203. Kurschner, C. and J.I. Morgan, *The cellular prion protein (PrP) selectively binds to Bcl-2 in the yeast two-hybrid system*. Brain Res Mol Brain Res, 1995. **30**(1): p. 165-8.
204. Bounhar, Y., et al., *Prion protein protects human neurons against Bax-mediated apoptosis*. J Biol Chem, 2001. **276**(42): p. 39145-9.
205. Kikuchi, Y., et al., *G1-dependent prion protein expression in human glioblastoma cell line T98G*. Biol Pharm Bull, 2002. **25**(6): p. 728-33.
206. Boison, D., et al., *Adhesive properties of proteolipid protein are responsible for the compaction of CNS myelin sheaths*. J Neurosci, 1995. **15**(8): p. 5502-13.
207. Klugmann, M., et al., *Assembly of CNS myelin in the absence of proteolipid protein*. Neuron, 1997. **18**(1): p. 59-70.

208. Kagawa, T., et al., *Glial cell degeneration and hypomyelination caused by overexpression of myelin proteolipid protein gene.* Neuron, 1994. **13**(2): p. 427-42.
209. Mallon, B.S. and W.B. Macklin, *Overexpression of the 3'-untranslated region of myelin proteolipid protein mRNA leads to reduced expression of endogenous proteolipid mRNA.* Neurochem Res, 2002. **27**(11): p. 1349-60.
210. Jiang, Z.Q., et al., *[Study of prognostic factors in patients with stage I non-small cell lung cancer].* Zhonghua Zhong Liu Za Zhi, 2004. **26**(6): p. 364-8.
211. Wight, P.A., et al., *A myelin proteolipid protein-LacZ fusion protein is developmentally regulated and targeted to the myelin membrane in transgenic mice.* J Cell Biol, 1993. **123**(2): p. 443-54.
212. Deak, F., et al., *The matrilins: a novel family of oligomeric extracellular matrix proteins.* Matrix Biol, 1999. **18**(1): p. 55-64.
213. Flower, D.R., *The lipocalin protein family: a role in cell regulation.* FEBS Lett, 1994. **354**(1): p. 7-11.
214. Boyles, J.K., L.M. Notterpek, and L.J. Anderson, *Accumulation of apolipoproteins in the regenerating and remyelinating mammalian peripheral nerve. Identification of apolipoprotein D, apolipoprotein A-IV, apolipoprotein E, and apolipoprotein A-I.* J Biol Chem, 1990. **265**(29): p. 17805-15.
215. Goodrum, J.F., et al., *Nerve regeneration and cholesterol reutilization occur in the absence of apolipoproteins E and A-I in mice.* J Neurochem, 1995. **64**(1): p. 408-16.
216. Peitsch, M.C., et al., *A purification method for apolipoprotein A-I and A-II.* Anal Biochem, 1989. **178**(2): p. 301-5.
217. Boyles, J.K., et al., *Identification, characterization, and tissue distribution of apolipoprotein D in the rat.* J Lipid Res, 1990. **31**(12): p. 2243-56.

218. Seguin, D., M. Desforges, and E. Rassart, *Molecular characterization and differential mRNA tissue distribution of mouse apolipoprotein D.* Brain Res Mol Brain Res, 1995. **30**(2): p. 242-50.

219. Simard, J., et al., *Additive stimulatory action of glucocorticoids and androgens on basal and estrogen-repressed apolipoprotein-D messenger ribonucleic acid levels and secretion in human breast cancer cells.* Endocrinology, 1992. **130**(3): p. 1115-21.

220. Provost, P.R., et al., *Apolipoprotein D transcription occurs specifically in nonproliferating quiescent and senescent fibroblast cultures.* FEBS Lett, 1991. **290**(1-2): p. 139-41.

221. Simard, J., et al., *Stimulation of apolipoprotein D secretion by steroids coincides with inhibition of cell proliferation in human LNCaP prostate cancer cells.* Cancer Res, 1991. **51**(16): p. 4336-41.

222. Dugoff, L. and E. Sujansky, *Neurofibromatosis type 1 and pregnancy.* Am J Med Genet, 1996. **66**(1): p. 7-10.

223. Lopez-Boado, Y.S., J. Tolivia, and C. Lopez-Otin, *Apolipoprotein D gene induction by retinoic acid is concomitant with growth arrest and cell differentiation in human breast cancer cells.* J Biol Chem, 1994. **269**(43): p. 26871-8.

224. Lopez-Boado, Y.S., et al., *Retinoic acid-induced expression of apolipoprotein D and concomitant growth arrest in human breast cancer cells are mediated through a retinoic acid receptor RARalpha-dependent signaling pathway.* J Biol Chem, 1996. **271**(50): p. 32105-11.

225. Rodriguez, J.C., et al., *Apolipoprotein D expression in benign and malignant prostate tissues.* Int J Surg Investig, 2000. **2**(4): p. 319-26.

226. Smits, A., et al., *Expression of platelet-derived growth factor and its receptors in proliferative disorders of fibroblastic origin.* Am J Pathol, 1992. **140**(3): p. 639-48.

227. Yeh, H.J., et al., *Developmental expression of the platelet-derived growth factor alpha-receptor gene in mammalian central nervous system.* Proc Natl Acad Sci U S A, 1993. **90**(5): p. 1952-6.
228. Yang, S.Y. and G.M. Xu, *Expression of PDGF and its receptor as well as their relationship to proliferating activity and apoptosis of meningiomas in human meningiomas.* J Clin Neurosci, 2001. **8 Suppl 1**: p. 49-53.

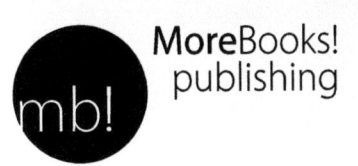
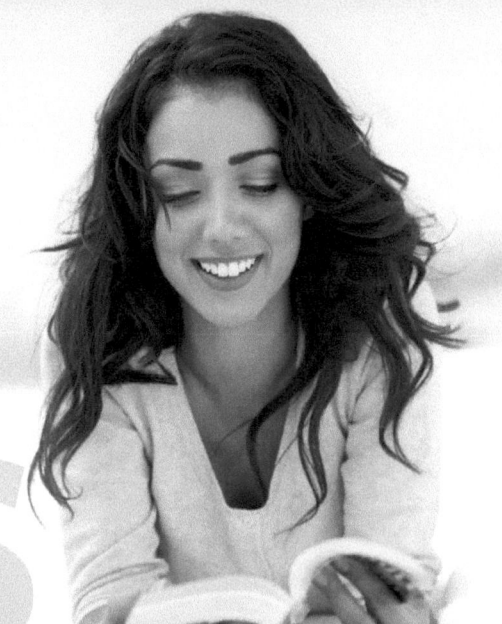

i want morebooks!

Buy your books fast and straightforward online - at one of world's fastest growing online book stores! Environmentally sound due to Print-on-Demand technologies.

Buy your books online at
www.get-morebooks.com

Kaufen Sie Ihre Bücher schnell und unkompliziert online – auf einer der am schnellsten wachsenden Buchhandelsplattformen weltweit! Dank Print-On-Demand umwelt- und ressourcenschonend produziert.

Bücher schneller online kaufen
www.morebooks.de

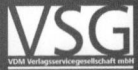

VDM Verlagsservicegesellschaft mbH
Heinrich-Böcking-Str. 6-8   Telefon: +49 681 3720 174   info@vdm-vsg.de
D - 66121 Saarbrücken   Telefax: +49 681 3720 1749   www.vdm-vsg.de

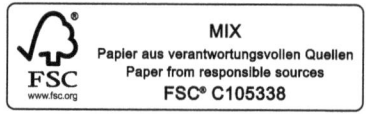

Printed by Books on Demand GmbH, Norderstedt / Germany